JO EAGER

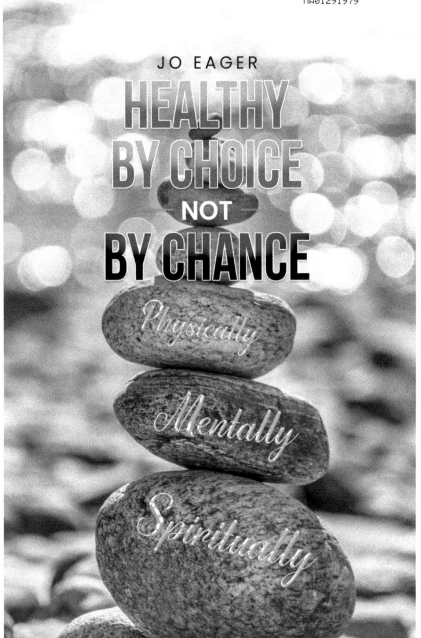

HEALTHY BY CHOICE NOT BY CHANCE

Physically

Mentally

Spiritually

outskirts
press

Outskirts Press, Inc.
http://www.outskirtspress.com

ISBN: 978-1-9772-5885-4

HEALTH DISCLAIMER
This book is about taking responsibility for your life, health, and safety at all times. The contents of this book are for educational and informational purposes.
There can be risk involved with exercise. The same is true with diet. Check with your physician before beginning changes to your diet and exercise program, especially if you have any medical conditions.

Outskirts Press and the "OP" logo are trademarks belonging to Outskirts Press, Inc.

PRINTED IN THE UNITED STATES OF AMERICA

"Jo's stories are riveting and enlightening. You can leap ahead in your spiritual growth, and enjoy the process more, simply by reading this book. You'll love it. I did. Expect Miracles!"

Dr Joe Vitale, author *"Zero Limits,"* star in *The Secret*

"In *Healthy by Choice, Not by Chance*, Jo talks directly to the person reading it, from a practical point of view. Jo gives her practical, personal examples of growth she experienced when facing personal challenges and the wisdom required to walk her talk. Jo begins with basic principles (your thinking) and moves gently into the physical realm of living life on life's terms. She includes spiritual lessons she has learned to assist her in maintaining a positive attitude about life.

Jo's views on the various aspects of health are very insightful. She explains how to turn adversities into opportunities. She uses her background and real experiences to reveal the underlying issues that both negative and positive thinking can create.

Her wealth of knowledge concerning weight, activity, and overall health comes from being a senior and her involvement in teaching Zumba® to seniors.

Insightful from beginning to end. I highly recommend it to anyone desiring to improve their health."

Michael McCright DD, HHP, CHC
Owner of "Together i Can"
"Where we encourage Pre-Hab over Re-Hab"
Prevention over Rehabilitation – Fix it Before it Happens

"Jo Eager's book reminded me of my purpose in life, in a light, upbeat, and researched way. Jo's personal experiences set a stage for her to teach us how to understand and apply the materials presented. It's packed with good ideas and suggestions. This is a joy to read."

Claire Levy, RN, Certified Reflexologist, and Reiki Master

"Taking responsibility for your life and making changes isn't easy. Let Jo Eager be the friend at your side helping you along the way. Sharing stories of her experiences and helpful advice is welcome, especially now when so many people feel alone."

Diane Ray, Host of the Podcast *Be Present: The Diane Ray Show*

May 2023

Better & Better!

Love,
Jo Lager

DEDICATION

This book is dedicated to you. And your health.

Table of Contents

Foreword

WHEN YOUR LONGTIME friend and soul sister asks you to write the foreword for her book, you say YES. That's been my motto for years…say YES to everything life brings you. Even when you don't know the *how-tos*, say yes and figure it out later. This "ask" was not only an honor, but a big yes, a *HELL YES!* Not only is Jo Eager a close and cherished friend, brilliant writer, news reporter, radio personality, voice over actor, mom, and seeker of the truth, but also a courageous soul, bright light, and spiritual teacher.

Her time has come. This book's time has come.

Jo and I met about 20 years ago at a weekly study group in San Diego. We studied "Concept Therapy," Dr. Thurman Fleet's philosophy on living life according to the natural laws of the body, mind, and soul, which was not only life-giving, but has been a spiritual beacon to light our path ever since. We included our kids, too. We were ALL IN. It's a philosophy that teaches how to live a better, more connected, healthier life through understanding and practicing the natural laws. God knows it helped us to have more faith. It was a sweet time of spiritual growth and community.

Jo and I instantly knew we were soul sisters (we looked alike, too) and supported each other in our life challenges from then on. We were grateful to have each other. We both had deep desires to share our growth and talents with the world in bigger ways.

We worked hard to *look for the good* as well as *get* the lessons. We made the best choices we could for where we were at the time, all the while continually studying and learning.

Life requires us to be brave enough to take risks sometimes, but when we do, doors open. Opportunities and possibilities come calling.

Jo did a variety of things over the years, including writing many published articles. She was eventually published in several *Chicken Soup for the Soul* books, an amazing accomplishment. She never stopped searching, looking for the synchronicities, or "divine thread" as I like to call it, for her next steps. When she found them (which she always would), she would say YES and move on.

In 2007, I lost my home to wildfire and two months later, was diagnosed with breast cancer. In 2008, Jo was bitten by a rattle-snake while hiking and in 2019, the news chopper she reported from (Chopper 8) crashed. In 2019, I collapsed with neuro-Lyme disease and 12 co-infections. These weren't small challenges, but potentially life-threatening ones.

We all have challenges, some worse than others. Is life going to stop throwing curve balls? No, but understand that your beliefs, self-talk, decisions, and actions (or inaction) create what you experience every day, especially during those turning point moments that can be so difficult to navigate.

If you believe life is happening TO you, life looks like it's against you. When you change your perception and realize life is happening FOR you, everything changes for the good. Neither Jo nor I believe things happen by chance. Even the craziest, scariest, most unfair events always give you the opportunity to gain understanding and compassion, express gratitude, and grow. You ALWAYS get to choose how you look at something, what you'll do with it (react or respond) and whether you'll grow from it.

In my experience, the Universe (God, the Great Something, Divine Energy) is always guiding us. If you look back over your life and explore your toughest moments, you'll see the synchronicities, divine orchestration, and people who showed up unexpectedly to help. The evidence/proof is always there, whether you choose to see and acknowledge it or not.

Why am I sharing all of this? I want you to know who Jo is and what she stands for. I want you to know she walks her talk and always has. She is a wonderful, sincere, loving human being with a huge heart, and I fully support her in bringing these amazing life stories and lessons straight to you. You will resonate with some of them and be touched by others. More importantly, if you take the nuggets and apply them to your own life, you will be forever changed.

If you are struggling in any way, this book is something you can hold onto. It's a powerful life guide created from life experiences, some extreme. It's honest and real. Within it are wonderful gems of wisdom. You can trust what's in this book because it's completely transparent. When you're reading, remember, Jo's stories are deeply personal and her insights profound. The real gift is that she gives you the pieces, the steps you need to shift your own life. This book came to be because someone genuinely cares about the quality of your life and happiness. Sometimes we need to learn lessons for ourselves. Sometimes we can take the shortcut and learn from other people's experiences.

I am so proud to call Jo Eager my friend. I'm elated she's finally releasing this book which comes from decades of the ups and downs in her life. All of it has been worthwhile because she has chosen to use it as a tool to help you.

Life will still throw you lemons sometimes, but how will you look at your experiences? What thoughts will you have? What choices will you make? How will you use what you've learned? Who will you be after you've moved through those experiences? Read this book, live it, and watch your world change for the better. The world needs awakened, hopeful, inspirational people now more than ever. Will you be a light for others?

Just say YES.

Lisa Winston
#1 Bestselling Author, Speaker, Artist and
Host of the *Mindset Reset TV Show*

Introduction

Choice: It is always your next move. ~ Napoleon Hill

CHOICE IS OUR greatest power. I've come to believe we create our world and are 100 percent responsible for our lives—whether experiencing health, peace, and happiness—or their opposites.

We wouldn't fill up a car's gas tank with water and expect it to run. The better the fuel, the better it runs. Same goes for our bodies, minds, and souls. What we ingest affects our performance. Making choices to eat healthy, exercise, think happy thoughts, and meditate, among many other decisions we make every day, make a difference in our overall health.

This book is based on my observations, research, opinions, and beliefs. It's a takeaway from my studies in health, wellness, exercise, nutrition, and universal laws. Some of these lessons changed my world.

It's easy to explain that it's important to drink enough water every day. It's a whole different story trying to explain how we create difficult conditions, circumstances, or events. I don't have answers to all of my questions, but I do have some that have been beneficial to me. Incorporate the ideas that resonate with you and leave the rest.

Even if we admit to creating our lives, it's not always obvious how some of our unwanted symptoms and circumstances came into being. For example, I have no idea how the pandemic that shut down the planet was "created." There were certainly global, as well as individual, lessons. During the quarantine, some cities saw blue skies for the first time in ages because there were very few motorists on the road. That was a good lesson for humanity: Quit abusing the universe. This could include changes to provide and use more efficient public transportation or have more people work from home, when possible, just to name a couple of ideas.

Our universe is not random. It operates lawfully and orderly, as can be seen in the phases of the moon, the tides of the ocean, the orbit of the planets, and the sun rising and setting at precise times.

Nothing happens by chance. Chance happenings would ensure total chaos. The universe would collapse. There are no coincidences, luck, or accidents. The law of cause and effect is always in operation, whether you believe it or not. It's like gravity. Even if you didn't believe in it, if you jump off a roof, you fall.

Everything is energy, including our thoughts and feelings. What you give out, you get back. There's opportunity to send loving vibrations that are met and returned by the same vibration. Choose honesty and you get back honesty. Put out fear, and fear comes back.

Change your thoughts and raise your frequency, and you change your world. Make a conscious choice to change a low vibration feeling of fear to a higher vibration of faith, even if it's just a little bit. You can do this by finding something positive, no matter how small, about the person, thing, or situation that's causing the fear or other negative feeling. If you're not happy with your life or some aspect of your life, my hope is that this book helps you make changes and choices to achieve peace and joy.

The greatest illusion in this world is the illusion of separation. ~ *Albert Einstein*

Quantum physicists and scientists recognize that everything in the universe is a manifestation of energy. We are connected and we are all One, from the same Source. From a religious perspective, God is omnipresent, everywhere at all times. With that in mind, the expression, "What you do unto your brother or sister, you do unto yourself," makes perfect sense.

What we observe as material bodies and forces are nothing but shapes and variations in the structure of space. Particles are just schaumkommen (appearances). ~ Erwin Schrodinger

Having this knowledge, we can learn to shift our energy, starting with our thoughts, feelings, and emotions. We can become more aware of our choices and how they impact our future, guiding us to a healthier life: physically, mentally, spiritually, and emotionally.

With knowledge, awareness, and a desire to take responsibility for our lives, we can consciously create the world of our dreams, as well as become healthier in every way.

CHAPTER 1

Comes a Time to Wake Up

WE ALL HAVE lessons and challenges in life. Some days they seem more like hassles and struggles. You've got to wonder sometimes— what's the purpose of an overflowing toilet or an invasion of termites? Do those count toward our growth—or is it just the biggies that count? Things like death, destruction, disease, divorce, and other tragedies. Being cool, calm, and collected when the pipes are clogged are admirable traits. But if you're like me, you sometimes find yourself cussing, mop in hand, as you clean up the bathroom floor.

While I believe we are responsible for our lives, I also believe everything happens for a reason. Experiences, both positive and negative, give us the opportunity to live, grow, and improve. Use your knowledge to figure out the reasons why certain things are happening. We may have wanted something, but it happened in an entirely different way than we ever could have imagined, and not always in ways we'd call "positive."

I've seen how major hardships have helped me evolve and become a better person; they've helped me to wake up. It's been a slow wake-up, my eyes opening a little more with each new challenge. Can a person experience trauma without an impact? Some people don't share the lessons learned or the growth they've experienced after riding down a rough road. They're still focusing on the challenge. For example, someone who had cancer and whose identity and life seem to revolve around being a "cancer survivor." Instead of telling the growth from the experience, the story is one of hardship and how bad it was. You may have to look for the good because it's not always obvious. What was the positive that came from it?

Others have taken their disadvantages and become teachers and mentors, offering inspiration. Wayne Dyer is a perfect example. The "Father of Motivation" never knew his dad, who abandoned the family shortly after Wayne's birth. He was in and out of foster homes and orphanages until his mother remarried. The new man in her life was an abusive alcoholic. Wayne learned early on to fend for himself. After his father's death, Wayne went to his dad's grave and was able to forgive him. He often spoke of how this transformed his life and motivated him to get off the road of self-destruction.

I was in a deep sleep when a few "earthquakes" started to shake me up and move me toward consciousness. My loved ones helped me along the path with their challenges, too.

Events Propelling Me Forward

Growing up, my dad was an alcoholic, but no one talked about it until we were older. I have three sisters and a brother, and I'm right in the middle. There were incidents you didn't really question since no one addressed them. Even with information, meetings, and literature available, if you're a kid and nobody at home is mentioning a problem, you don't question what's happening.

For example, one afternoon when my younger sister and I came home from elementary school, our dad was passed out on the kitchen floor. The kitchen was not very big, and we had to step over him to get a snack. We didn't even say anything to each other, like: "Wow, this is weird—Dad sprawled out on the kitchen floor." So we grew up thinking, "This is normal."

Dad was not a mean drunk, but sometimes he'd forget about "promises" because of his drinking. We were either left in a bind if the promise was to help us with something or left feeling unimportant because he didn't show up to do whatever it was that he'd promised.

As teenagers, we sometimes gave Dad a hard time about his drinking. He'd tell us he only planned to live to be 60. In his mid-to-late 50s, he upped it to 65 because 60 was rapidly approaching. He made it to 64.

What are the benefits of alcoholism? The 12 Steps.

In my early twenties, I visited and loved the beauty of the Ozarks. That was a good enough reason for me to move from South Dakota to Arkansas. Meanwhile, my mom and a couple of my sisters started attending Al-Anon meetings. They sent me Al-Anon literature, but I had no interest at the time. After all, I thought, I'm not around my dad that much anymore.

I was working as a radio disc jockey and bounced around to a few different jobs, towns, and relationships. I ended up moving back to South Dakota about five years later after an abusive relationship.

During my job search at radio stations in Sioux Falls, I visited a U.S. Army Reserve recruiting office. My intention was to inquire about becoming a weekend warrior. I enlisted. Fulltime. No weekend business. I didn't even take a day to think about it. My rationale: I'll never be able to travel the world on DJ pay so why not sign up?

More Steps Forward

After training, I was stationed in Berlin, Germany. At first, living in a foreign country was rather surreal for me; getting to know a culture, city, language, and so much more. I ended up staying for 10 years.

Two years after moving to Berlin, I began going to 12 Step meetings after meeting my husband, a recovering alcoholic. Now I had an interest in the 12 Steps and attended Al-Anon regularly. I also checked out Adult Children of Alcoholics (ACOA). For me, and so many others, it's a spiritual program that helped me connect more deeply with God. Practicing the steps aided me in becoming a better person. I evolved as I took a step, or rather 12, forward.

CHAPTER 2

Behind the Iron Curtain

(Originally published in *Chicken Soup for the Soul: Military Families*)

History studies not just facts and institutions; its real subject is the human spirit. ~ *Numa Denis Fustel de Coulanges*

IT WAS COLD and gray when I arrived in Frankfurt, Germany, in December 1981. A few days later, I received my orders for the American Forces Network (AFN), Berlin— 101 miles behind the Iron Curtain.

After working a few years as a radio disc jockey as a teenager, I joined the Army to use my broadcast experience to entertain the troops—and to travel the world. I hadn't envisioned Berlin, a divided city during the Cold War. West Berlin was an island in the middle of East Germany, and following World War II it was occupied by the United States, France, and England; East Berlin was occupied by Russia.

For soldiers traveling from Frankfurt to West Berlin, it was an overnight ride through East Germany on the Army duty train. "Flag orders" were issued with one's name, rank, and personal information.

At the train station before boarding, a loudspeaker blared rules for duty train travel through the East: no photography, no looking out the windows, which had shades pulled down, no throwing anything out the windows, no exiting the train when it stopped at checkpoints in East Germany, and no conversing or making eye contact with any Soviet or East German personnel.

The train's sleeping cars had bunks, so one could sleep during the ten-hour ride. At some point during the journey, I just had to sneak a peek out the window. It was pitch black, and I couldn't see a thing. When we stopped at a station, I could see lights and a few people in uniform on the platform as I discreetly peered out the small space between the shade and the window.

Arriving in West Berlin, a woman from my unit was there to greet me. After a quick rundown at our barracks, she showed me to my room. A life very different from what I was used to in the United States began.

In addition to learning my job responsibilities that first day, one of my new colleagues asked me to a concert that night. He'd interviewed the performer earlier in the week and had free tickets.

Unpacking could wait. I wanted to take in as much of this new, strange place as I could.

My new adventure was underway as we rode the U-Bahn (underground subway) to get to the venue. I learned how to read the map and buy a ticket for the U-Bahn, and how to count to ten in German.

After the concert, we met up with German friends of my colleague. I learned a little more German, had my first taste of Apfelkorn (a German liqueur made with apples), and made new friends, who warmly welcomed me with their laughter and stories.

I enrolled in German classes, practicing what I learned at stores and eateries. As an added and unexpected bonus, I married two years later. My husband, an Air Force sergeant I met through work, had two children; a year later, we had another one.

I met Germans who loved and appreciated Americans and enjoyed telling their stories. Others protested with anti-American demonstrations.

Along with strudel and sauerkraut, plenty of stress was served. One day, we had a bomb threat at AFN. We were given notice to evacuate, but first we had to check our work area for a bomb. I had no idea what a bomb looked like, but looked around for any strange object. Turns out, a bomb was found at the bottom of one of our transmitters located at a different site.

On April 5, 1986, there was a large explosion at the La Belle nightclub in Berlin, well known as a popular American hangout. Two U.S. soldiers and a Turkish woman were killed. The blast injured 230 people, including more than seventy American service members.

The following Monday, a co-worker, noticeably shaken, told me he'd been at La Belle that night, leaving shortly before the bomb went off. He realized it could have been him and felt relief, yet grief.

Tension followed as the U.S. retaliated. My kids evacuated school due to a bomb threat. School buses had machine-gun escorts. We were told to check under our vehicles for bombs before turning the key in the ignition. Things eventually quieted down.

In 1987, President Reagan celebrated America's birthday party for Berlin. After his speech at the Brandenburg Gate, he visited the American Air Force base. Three stages were set up for entertainment before he arrived, and I was honored when asked to emcee one of those stages.

After leaving the military, my husband and I stayed in West Berlin, working for a German radio station founded after World War II. Target audience: East Berlin and East Germany, giving them a view of the news from a western perspective. Many tuned in, although it was forbidden for them to listen.

After ground war broke out in Iraq in 1991, my husband and I were taken off the air as a security measure. The kids went to a German-American school, and it was canceled, so they were home, too. I was concerned about them going to any American institutions, but pretty much everything closed for a short while, even the American church.

The night my husband was back on the air, there was a bomb threat at the radio station. He also received some threatening letters. Fortunately, none turned out to be real.

My house was located a half-mile from Potsdam, East Germany. The Berlin Wall was a chain-link fence in this area, so when I jogged near no-man's land, I watched East German guards patrolling, sitting in a tower or driving an Army jeep on a narrow-paved strip. I never thought I'd see the day I'd be riding a bike or jogging on that strip.

On November 9, 1989, the most exciting news came. The East German government announced that restrictions on travel and emigration had ended. I witnessed the fall of the Iron Curtain and the Berlin Wall. As a journalist, I helped print and broadcast media in the U.S. get interviews and do translations.

A refugee camp was set up near my house. I visited regularly, looking for English speakers for interviews. Many told their stories about leaving the East to make a new life in the West. I still have contact with some of the people I befriended during that time.

I joined the military to travel and see the world. If I hadn't joined the Army, I never would have gone to Berlin and stayed for ten years. My travels during that time took me to twenty countries. One weekend, I was invited as a guest DJ at a discotheque in Poland—what a dancing frenzy. I rode a camel in Morocco and went camping near Prague.

It was a wonderful opportunity with many unique, interesting, and tremendous experiences. Had I been asked where I wanted to be stationed, I'd have picked skiing the slopes of Stuttgart or Munich. Glad they didn't ask. If my orders had taken me anywhere else, I would've missed out personally with my firstborn child and historically with a monumental event that, to this day, gives me chills when I say… "I was there."

CHAPTER **3**

When the Wind Blows

BY THE TIME the calendar hit the 1990s, any passion for both my marriage and living in Germany was non-existent. After months of mental debate, I made the extremely difficult decision to move with my child back to the U.S., leaving my husband and step-kids behind. I wanted to be near family, so I moved near one of my sisters on Kauai, Hawaii.

During this time, reading Louise Hay's book, *You Can Heal Your Life*, was an inspiration. It's had a major impact on me, and I reread it regularly. Reinforcement of the concepts Hay shares comes to me regularly through numerous other books I've read.

One year into living in paradise, Hurricane Iniki paid a visit. We were left with no electricity, no water, no local radio, no phones (and this was before cell phones). It was a category four hurricane that hit the island with a vengeance, sustained winds at 145 miles per hour, gusting to 175. We were all left totally isolated from the rest of the world with no clue of what was even happening on other parts of the island. It was one of the most destructive hurricanes to strike Hawaii.

It started with sirens blaring around 5:30 the morning of Friday, September 11, 1992. I turned on the radio. No school. The mayor wanted everyone off the streets by 10:30. Strong winds would start at 1:00 that afternoon, and the eye of the hurricane would reach us at about 5:00. People waited in lines at gas stations for up to three hours. Shoppers crowded stores buying batteries, water, charcoal, and canned food. Houses were boarded up.

My hurricane prep: I filled containers and the bathtub with water; showered and shaved while we still had water; used the curling iron while we still had electricity. I was ready for a date with Iniki. Before leaving the house, I cracked the windows just right, hoping the hurricane wouldn't destroy them. I turned off the electricity and headed to my sister's a few miles away. We cooked the food that was in the freezer. There were five of us: my sister, our friend and her daughter, and me and my child. At 1:30, we huddled in a small hallway with pillows and soft cushions surrounding us.

The kids had instructions on "take cover"—rolling over with faces to the floor, pillow and arms protecting their heads. The winds grew stronger by the minute. We listened to the radio until the station lost power, as well as its generator. Looking out the window, I observed pieces of the neighbor's roof flying by. It was like a bad scene from the Wizard of Oz. The lattices blew from the carport, standing erect in the middle of the yard by the power of the wind. The thought of winds getting stronger terrified me. We prayed. It became so intense it seemed the entire island, with everyone on it, might blow away.

Time dragged as we anxiously awaited 5:00. Finally, as predicted, the winds changed. During the eye of the hurricane, we took a look outside. The avocado tree was overturned. The lattices and other objects from the carport had blown across the yard. By 6:30, after five hours in that hallway with only a few breaks, it was over, we were alive, and my sister's house and roof were in place. It was still blowing, but later that night, it became eerily still.

The following morning, we drove first to our friend's house to check out the damage—a screen and glass door had blown off, but the glass didn't break. There were broken jalousies and the skylight on the guest house was broken. Debris covered the front yard consisting of portions of the neighbor's house and roof.

Next stop was my house. What a strange feeling driving down your street anxiously waiting to see if your house is still standing and, if so, with a roof. Driving up, it looked good. The deck's three glass French doors were intact. With a third of the roof gone, several rooms were soaked. We immediately found a tarp and covered the roof.

Dodging wires and telephone poles, we toured Poipu. With no electricity, resorts were grilling food, offering it free to everyone. It was strange to see the lack of green around the island. Branches and leaves were everywhere. Many trees were uprooted. The "tree tunnel" became the "twig tunnel."

What a blessing the full moon was those first nights as we adapted to life without electricity and lights.

A couple of days after the hurricane, we started cleaning up our yards—and then ourselves. The five of us went to the Botanical Gardens stream to bathe. The water was cold, but we squealed in delight at how glorious it felt to get cleaned up.

I purchased a couple of new garbage cans to take to the fire department where they filled them up with water. The local radio station was back on the air. With battery-operated radios, we could now get information. Free military flights were available for tourists and others wanting to get off the island. Knowing Mom would be worried, we stopped by the airport and asked a tourist to call her once they got to Honolulu.

Surveying the island showed a grim picture with so many homes demolished. The island was devastated, a total disaster area—it looked like a war zone. The national guard fit right in. Everyone was affected. It was unbelievable the amount of damage done in just five hours—$1.8 billion. Recovery, reconstruction, and rebuilding would take a long time. Our former lives no longer existed. It was a true test of trust. There were tears but also moments knowing that everything would be okay.

Two and a half weeks later, schools reopened on a limited schedule without electricity. When stores eventually opened, you could only buy necessities. A store employee escorted shoppers, one at a time, with a flashlight. Long lines waited at gas stations. Trauma teams arrived. Seven emergency centers popped up around the island. Special coloring books helped kids deal with the disaster. Free flights were offered to kids if parents wanted to send them to live with relatives on other islands. Emergency centers and churches had free supplies: candles, Coleman stoves, batteries, food items, gas canisters. Phone banks were set up so everyone could call loved ones around the world. These became more than just phone banks, though. In addition to connecting afar, they became social places where people gathered to find out how friends and neighbors were doing.

Without electricity, I hurriedly washed the dishes before dark. We rushed to do everything before dark—like get home. It was enough of a challenge driving during the day dodging wires and telephone and electric poles all over the roads. I picked up ice on a regular basis—our refrigeration. My friend had a gas hot water heater, so we'd go to her place to shower. No doing laundry. We went to Molokai for a few days just to get away and packed dirty clothes.

It was four weeks before power was restored to my house—at that point I was in the 20 percent of those so fortunate. Some people waited six months. When I got home that day, I flipped the switches—lights went on, fridge hummed—it was absolutely magnificent. I took a hot shower, turned on the stereo, played music, emptied out my shower bag that I kept ready to take with me to catch a hot shower at a friend's, and emptied the several coolers in the garage I'd accumulated. I set the electric clock, turned the word processor on, and started writing. The next morning, I savored my first pot of coffee at home in four weeks. This was the life of luxury. Absolutely wonderful. I did laundry, washing everything I could find, vacuumed, and cleaned the house.

During the aftermath of Iniki, people got to know their neighbors better. There's nothing like disaster to bring about camaraderie—coming together to get through an event with a common goal—rebuilding Kauai. People helping people. I spent many hours helping clean up houses. My neighbors had a Coleman stove and invited us over for meals. One morning breakfast was lamb chops, potatoes, and coffee. The neighborhood center, another place to meet up with or make new friends, offered meals, in addition to military MREs (Meals Ready to Eat) to take home. Gratitude was abundant—so many simple pleasures to be grateful for that we often take for granted.

CHAPTER 4

The World was Turned Upside Down

REBUILDING THE ISLAND began with numerous construction companies from the mainland. That's when I met my younger child's father, which led to my move to San Diego. When the relationship dissolved a couple of years after the baby was born, I became a single mom with a toddler and a teenager.

I was working in radio and television, the little one started preschool, and the older one was in high school, eventually graduating and moving out to attend college—accumulating three degrees in a nine-year period: Juris Doctorate, a Master's in Business Administration, and a Bachelor's in Political Science.

Then, in 2002, my world was turned upside down.

Originally published in *Chicken Soup for the Soul: Find Your Inner Strength*

Bag of Hope

There is no hope unmingled with fear, and no fear unmingled with hope. ~ Baruch Spinoza

It was five o'clock on a Friday afternoon when Nathan came to the door. His blond hair was cut short; his blue eyes matched the warmth of his smile. It was his eighth birthday.

Instead of receiving gifts, he was bringing them. He brought with him his parents, his younger brother, and on his shoulder he carried a Bag of Hope.

My six-year-old son, Kaipo, greeted them at the door.

"Show Kaipo what's in the Bag of Hope," said Nathan's father.

The boy spilled the contents of the bag onto the couch. He didn't save the best for last. He started with the best, a teddy bear named Rufus.

"I sleep with mine every night," Nathan told Kaipo.

Rufus, the Bear with Diabetes, comes complete with a medical identification bracelet to show that he has diabetes and patches on his body to show where he takes insulin shots: his arms, legs, abdomen and buttocks.

"I give Rufus shots, just like I have to take," said Nathan.

He went through the rest of the items in the Bag of Hope, giving some to Kaipo and some to me—kids' books, coloring books, a video, and some literature for parents.

Then he took out his blood testing kit and showed Kaipo how he tests blood from his arm instead of his fingertips.

Earlier that day, Nathan's father had called me to set up a time to meet. The Juvenile Diabetes Research Foundation had hooked them up with my son and me.

Nathan had been diagnosed with type 1 diabetes six months earlier, his father told me.

"When was your son diagnosed?" he asked.

"Two weeks ago," I said.

"You must be a basket case."

He understood. Here was someone who could actually relate to me in a way that others couldn't.

"Yes," I told him. "Sometimes I just start crying in the middle of a conversation."

He knew the fear I felt, the grief, the sadness, the loss. He could identify with my pain.

It was amazing how much life had changed overnight. Suddenly I was a nurse checking my son's blood at least four times a day, giving him shots of insulin twice a day, making sure he had the right amount of food to eat six times a day. I dropped my son off at school with worries that were so magnified from what they'd been just days ago.

Would my son know if his blood sugar level was too low? I recited the symptoms over and over to him.

Our three-day stay in the hospital had been intense. It was a crash course in diabetes, and it was overwhelming. I knew that once we got home, I wouldn't have the nurses there to answer my questions. I was on my own. What if I couldn't remember something I'd learned over the past few days? I didn't have the other parent in the home to help me remember all the information that had poured into my brain.

My worry was constant and extreme. That's the part of single parenting that I find the hardest—taking on 100 percent of the fear and stress of the situation. The other parent isn't there to take on half of it. Nathan's mom said she worried about her son's blood sugar level getting too high. His dad worried more if it got too low. I worried about both, but was more scared of hypoglycemia (low blood sugar). It happens quickly and can lead to unconsciousness. If it became low in his sleep, would he wake up?

Parents like Nathan's say, "Call anytime," and they mean it. They let me know that I'm normal.

"It was bedtime and his reading was low. I gave him extra carbohydrates and had him sleep in my bed."

"We've all done that."

When I first called JDRF, the woman I spoke with told me, "I cried every day for three months after my child was diagnosed." With time, the tears eventually dry, replaced with experience and knowledge.

Nathan's Bag of Hope brought more than its contents. With it came experience, kindness and sympathy. I'd heard that most parents say it takes them a year to feel comfortable with their child's diabetes. Just six months into their own son's diagnosis, Nathan's parents were out offering support—that alone gave me a lot of hope.

That evening after I gave Kaipo his shot of insulin, he took the used syringe and gave Rufus a shot. As a matter of fact, Rufus had several shots that night. It must have been the right dose—he slept peacefully in Kaipo's arms all night. The dose of hope was just right, too—Kaipo's been holding that teddy bear tight every night since, just like Nathan.

If it's true that in giving we receive, Nathan had the best birthday ever.

That was the event that really got me started on the road to gaining knowledge on health, wellbeing, the laws of the universe and of the body, mind, and soul.

CHAPTER 5

What are You Creating?

JUST LIKE THAT, I became a nurse overnight. I was overwhelmed with all the information I needed to know in order to keep my son's blood sugar in balance. I wasn't consciously looking for any teachings or programs, but one magazine article took me on a journey of evolution and awareness that changed my life. I discovered Concept-Therapy, a philosophy to help create a better life with more health, happiness, and peace. I learned about the laws of the body, mind, soul, and universe, and how they affect my life. Change your concepts, change your life. The philosophy brings theology and science together, along with metaphysics, psychology, and sociology.

My thoughts, feelings, emotions, words, and actions matter. Like everything, they vibrate.

Notice things you say and what others say to you. What are you listening to? Observe the media, gossip, everyday expressions, and negative self-talk.

Listening to the news, which covers so much drama, destruction, disease, and disaster in a hyped-up mode is mostly negative. Beating yourself up and telling yourself things like, "I'm so fat" or "Why did I say something so stupid?" are obviously not nice ways to talk to yourself. It takes effort, but these thoughts can be stopped. Think before you speak is a great message, but no one does it 24/7 for their entire life. We've all had times we've regretted something we've said.

We're all works in progress. The important thing is to work toward becoming a better, more evolved person.

We're creators. When you don't take responsibility for what's happening in your life and believe that things just happen or it's someone else's fault, you're giving your power away. The law of cause and effect is always at work. What you sow is what you reap—sow positive seeds and reap the constructive things of life. Choose positive mental states such as charity, courage, love, and compassion, and you align yourself with Spirit. When you find yourself dwelling on the negative aspects of worry, fear, and hate, cancel those thoughts and replace them with their opposites. Just like when you plant tomatoes—your garden grows tomatoes, not cucumbers.

When I catch myself having undesirable thoughts, I immediately think or say out loud, "Cut, cancel, delete." This helps stop the negative thoughts and get rid of them.

Keep in mind that when you ask for something, as in "I want...," in order for the Universe to grant it, you're kept in a state of wanting. Instead, assume the feeling of the wish fulfilled.

Stay away from researching symptoms. As an example, let's say you're headed toward the age of menopause. You get online and start researching symptoms others have experienced. Next thing you know, as you reach menopause, you start developing some of the symptoms you read about, such as hot flashes. When I went through menopause, I don't recall having any "symptoms" other than not getting my monthly period. No complaints there.

Putting these Lessons to the Test

LET'S PRACTICE. LET'S SAY YOU'RE WORRIED ABOUT SOMETHING.

Apply constructive thought. Use this thought to determine if the situation can be changed or solved. If it's not in your power to work out the problem, refuse to worry about it. I've had many times where I've found it extremely difficult, often in the middle of the night, to stop my mind from going to worst-case scenarios. It takes discipline. Whatever the situation is, picture everything working out. Pray. Repeat a mantra. Read something inspirational. Call a friend (well, maybe not in the middle of the night).

Practice faith. When you're thinking and feeling fear, replace it with faith. It takes practice. Lots of it. Replace negative emotions with their opposites. We all know people who rub us the wrong way. Try sending them white light and love. There's a 20-something-year-old guy in my neighborhood whose behavior is troublesome. I send him white light and love. It's not an immediate response for me to pray for him, but eventually, I do. It can't hurt.

Get rid of anger. Instead, practice patience. Positive, constructive emotions can dilute, neutralize, and overcome the negative.

By studying, learning, and practicing the laws of the Universe and making the right choices for your body, mind, and soul, you can deliberately and consciously choose to bring your life into harmony with the Divine.

A desire to be healthy means thinking, talking, and acting healthy. When you talk, you create your world. Choose uplifting thoughts, words, and actions. What is it you want? Think, talk, and act according to how you answered that question. If you desire financial abundance, don't talk about lack and how broke you are. Look at areas where you are abundant and give gratitude for what you already have. Do you have plenty of food in the refrigerator? Do you have lots of good friends? Give thanks. Be grateful always. Where attention goes, energy flows.

A key to succeeding with this effort of watching our words goes back to awareness and training ourselves to respond, not react. It would become exhausting to be on guard with every word that comes out of our mouths, but really paying attention to our feelings can be a big help. When someone says something that makes you defensive, it's a challenge to think before blurting out whatever comes to mind, which can be harmful.

To create health in your life, talk about health, not ailments and diseases. Hang out with like-minded people.

Let's Walk for Health—or is it Dis-ease?

Disease is big business. There are "walks" for almost every kind of disease. While the intention is for a cure, there's a lot of focus put on the disease itself, along with the survivors and their stories, all of it centering on the disease. Yes, they do talk about hope, too, but the attention is still on the illness. In addition, it's called a war or battle against the disease, which means resistance. Resistance puts you out of harmony with Source Energy.

Keep the slogan in mind, "What you resist persists." Resist nothing. Fighting against things is resistance, and there's a lot of that going on. The "fight" against all kinds of diseases, the "battle" of the bulge, "struggling" with whatever illness, "fighting" for his/her life—the list goes on. They're all words of resistance.

There are entire months dedicated to disease awareness. I'd rather be aware of health, wouldn't you?

When you're in harmony and living joyfully, the Universe moves to fulfill your thoughts. When you resist what is, you disconnect yourself from Spirit Energy, and inspiration can't flow. When you lose that connection, you start to experience things like illness. Fighting and pushing against what you don't want or like can create friction, which can create disharmony in your body. Choose what you do want.

The money raised on walks for disease does go toward terrific advancements, thanks to research, but here's some food for thought when it comes to finding a cure:

It is difficult to get a man to understand something, when his salary depends upon his not understanding it. ~ Upton Sinclair.

A cure would make a lot of jobs unnecessary.

Also, when it comes to enlisting in the war against your cause, keep this in mind from author, journalist, and speaker Phillip Day:

Wars are only profitable while you are fighting them, not when you've won them. That's right. Welcome to the not-so-enchanted forest of baleful scientific endeavor. Cancer is a $200 billion-a-year industry. There are more people today making a living from cancer than there are dying from it. 'From an economic point of view alone,' one professor confided, 'why would anyone ever wish to cure cancer? Millions would have to re-train.'

What about Genes?

In his extensive teachings and writings, stem-cell biologist and best-selling author Dr. Bruce Lipton explains that we are not powerless over our health, and we can literally change the fate of our cells by altering our thoughts. (His website is www.brucelipton.com.) Control is not in the genes, but it's our environment and our perceptions that control genetics. With that being the case, he says, we can be a master by changing our beliefs, perceptions, and environment, which in turn, changes your genetics. In his book *The Biology of Belief: Unleashing the Power of Consciousness, Matter and Miracles*, he notes:

We are not victims of our genes, but masters of our fates, able to create lives overflowing with peace, happiness, and love.

CHAPTER 6

Making a Difference

IF YOU'RE EVER unsure of what action to take, ask yourself if it's good for you. If it is, what about others—is the action beneficial to others or harmful? If it's beneficial, consider the effect your action will have on everyone and everything—all that exists.

Recognizing that all of life—everything and everyone—is the same energy vibrating at different frequencies, it's easy to understand that our actions will have an impact on others.

Some people who've had near-death experiences say that during the time they were dead, they became aware of everything and everyone being connected and how everything we do affects not only the people involved but the entire universe.

You never know how much your words or actions can change another person's life, both in a good way or a not-so-good way. Just a few words of praise can change a child's world. They may have been ready to give up until a little bit of encouragement renewed their spirit.

Have you heard of Helice "Sparky" Bridges, a teacher in New York? She honored all of her students, letting each of them know, individually, how they made a difference to her and to the class. She then gave each of them a blue ribbon that said, "Who I Am Makes a Difference." As a class project, she then gave each student three blue ribbons to pass along to someone they felt deserved one, and that person took the other two ribbons to pass along. One boy honored a junior executive who helped him in his career planning. He put a blue ribbon on the man's shirt, then gave him the other two blue ribbons to pass along. The junior executive chose his boss, a bit of a grumpy fellow, to honor with a ribbon. In addition, the boss was given the last blue ribbon to pass along. When the boss got home, he told his 14-year-old son about the "Who You Are Makes a Difference" ribbon he'd received, then gave his son a blue ribbon, letting the boy know how important he was in his father's life. The boy broke down in tears, telling his father he had planned to commit suicide that night and had just finished writing a note to his parents. What a tremendous impact this "school project" had on their lives.

When I was a teenager and just out of high school, I moved to a town an hour south of my hometown. My job search took me to the local newspaper where I hoped to get a position as a writer. A friend of my mom's casually mentioned an opening at the local radio station, so I put in an application. The next 46 years I spent in radio and television and worked at stations from Berlin, Germany, to Kauai, Hawaii, along with several places in-between. I had found my passion all because of a few words from a woman I'd just met.

Doing the right thing means evolution for you and all of Consciousness.

If your body is having issues, allow well-being and let the healing begin. You can do this by accepting things just the way they are. Your body knows what to do. If you cut yourself, the body quickly forms a scab and goes to work to heal it. Instead of fighting, embrace prayer, meditation, and visualization. Knowing that the body is an effect, take time to figure out the cause.

Creating Neural Pathways

Merriam-Webster defines neural pathways as a series of connected nerves along which electrical impulses travel in the body. They send signals from one part of the brain to another. Continually having the same thoughts, beliefs, habits, and concepts reinforces them, regardless of whether they're beneficial to us. If a person always smokes a cigarette after a meal, it becomes automatic. This can all be changed by switching those thoughts or habits to something more positive, creating more positive pathways and decreasing the negative. When you eventually have more of the positive energy than the negative, your brain will automatically choose positive thoughts more often than negative ones.

I read a story about a woman over the age of 40 who decided to learn to ice skate. She learned new tricks on the ice and practiced them over and over, getting a little bit better each time. In addition to repeating the moves, she felt her focused attention also helped develop new neural pathways.

We can rewire our brains. As we process new information, neurons fire and new pathways are created. This happens throughout our lifetimes when we give the brain new material to practice.

With awareness, start noticing when thoughts start to travel down an unwanted path and consciously choose to change them. Easier said than done. It takes time and discipline to make it a habit and retrain the brain. But you can learn to control your mind, allowing only positive, desirable thoughts.

A study at the University College of London showed it takes an average of approximately 66 days of repetition for a new habit to take form, indicating a change in the neural pathway.

Many people have heard that it takes 21 days to change a behavior. According to an article by James Clear (https://james-clear.com/new-habit), this 21-day idea came from Dr. Maxwell Maltz back in the 1950s. Through observations in his work, Dr. Maltz found and wrote, "These, and many other commonly observed phenomena tend to show that it requires a minimum of about 21 days for an old mental image to dissolve and a new one to jell."

Clear went on to say that many professionals have since used the 21-day information but without the word "minimum." He tells about a study on changing habits that showed it typically takes more than two months for new behaviors to become automatic.

The exact number will vary, "depending on the behavior, the person, and the circumstances." In the study, the range was from 18 days to 254 days.

Be patient with yourself. You can change.

CHAPTER 7

Mindset has Everything to Do with It

WHILE MANY OF the teachings in this book are simple, they're not always easy; for example, replacing worry with hope. My mind—oh, how it tends to veer off in some of the most negative directions.

"Will I have enough money for the extra work needed on the house?"

"Why isn't my son home yet? Where is he? Is he okay?"

Negative thoughts do not attract positivity into our lives, and they create negative vibrations.

Charles Haanel wrote in *The Master Key System*: "Nothing can reach us except what is necessary for our growth. All conditions and experiences come to us for our benefit. Difficulties and obstacles will continue to come only until we absorb their wisdom and gather from them the essentials for further growth."

There is a Divine plan. When you have a situation or circumstance that causes you hopelessness or despair, see it as an opportunity to use your strength to gain victory over the hardship. From that challenge, you evolve and grow.

Sometimes, as the plan unfolds, what at first appears as a "bad" thing may bring you more "good" than you ever imagined.

The singer/songwriter Adele went through a painful breakup. She channeled her energy into writing songs about the breakup and won several Grammy awards. It turned out to be a very productive breakup with some outstanding and wonderful benefits.

Different situations are viewed in various ways. For example, during a war, some consider it okay to kill. Yet, if they did that to their neighbor, it would not be okay. Others view war as big business and enjoy hefty profits.

When someone is hurting, we feel sadness, pain, and compassion. To uplift, it's important to move on to seeing that person overcoming their challenge. Picture the person the way you want them to be—healthy and happy. Bless them with your good and positive thoughts and vibrations.

Many successes have come from people's difficulties. Suffering is responsible for some of the most profound contributions to society.

Remember, you get what you think about most of the time. Keeping that in mind, how do you view things such as success or failure? Thomas Edison was asked about his failures when trying to create the light bulb. His response was, "I have not failed. I've just found 10,000 ways that won't work." He understood that every time he found a way that didn't work, he was ultimately getting closer to success.

Even with a lot of knowledge, we are living among, and surrounded by, many people who have no clue regarding the laws of the universe and the Oneness of Life. Their actions, especially the ones we call bad, might affect us. How can we meet such a situation without reacting or making a choice not to let it bother us? Start by choosing friends who are living on the positive side of life, who always try to do the right thing. Avoid negative people who all too often make the wrong choices.

If you meet people who do something that affects you in a negative way, try to keep your outlook positive, knowing that with the law of cause and effect they will reap what they sow and get their just reward— without you doing anything (other than keeping your focus on the positive).

If you're making a conscious effort to keep your thoughts positive, as well as doing and saying what you consider the right things but you're having a down day, remember that if you continue to keep your mind focused on the good, the downer mood will pass more swiftly. There is rhythm throughout the Universe. Full moon, new moon. High tide, low tide. Just like our emotions—high and low.

Enjoy the peace, harmony, and contentment that accompany positive emotions, such as generosity, aspiration, kindness, sympathy, and love. Ride out the days when you're feeling worry, fear, criticism, or anger. It's true—this too shall pass. Hard as it may be, keep your mind coming back to gratitude. That'll help the lows move out more quickly.

Situations and circumstances that at first seem negative often, if not always, have a bright side. We may have to look for it.

Where Was my Mind when I Attracted This?

I've had many times I've asked myself: How did I bring that into my life? One of those incidents was in 2008 when I was given the opportunity to seek out the gift from a life-threatening situation that was a painful, horrible nightmare. I spent fifteen days in the hospital and five to six weeks recovering and learning to walk again after being temporarily paralyzed.

Here's the story:

Rattled
(Originally published in *Chicken Soup for the Soul: From Lemons to Lemonade*)

The deafening sound of the rescue helicopter sliced the still, spring air. The chopper got into position, lowered and hovered over a San Diego hilltop, dropping a member of a rescue crew to the ground. I'd seen this scene unfold many times in my career as an airborne news and traffic reporter. This time, though, was different. I was the person being rescued! They lifted me to the harness. I was hoisted—dangling in the air—to the waiting aircraft. The chopper flew me to an ambulance waiting nearby. Then one of the most difficult journeys of my life began.

It all started earlier that afternoon as I set off to hike my favorite trail. About a half-hour into the hike, a short portion of the path became very narrow, covered with thick, waist-high grass. I knew the trail well so I always scurried quickly through this part since I couldn't see what might be lurking. Making fast tracks, I suddenly heard a rattle. Like an antelope racing from a cheetah, I turned around and ran as fast as I could to reach my hiking buddy, JP, who was a bit of a distance behind me.

"I heard a rattlesnake," I gasped

He eyed my bloody ankle. "I'll call 911."

"No, I'm okay. I hit a branch or something." I said, annoyed that he'd want to freak me out.

"Okay." He flipped his cell phone shut.

My ankle did hurt—it felt like someone had hammered thorns into my leg. Despite the fact that I'd heard a rattle, I was in denial that a snake had bitten me. It didn't take long to grasp the situation, though. Within 10 seconds, my hands and fingers were tingling and numb.

"Call 911," my voice shook.

JP stayed on the phone, giving directions as we waited for the helicopter.

"Keep the heart above the injury and don't panic," JP said, repeating what the person on the other end of the phone said. *Don't panic?!* I felt my insides swelling. My breathing was labored and difficult. Closing my eyes, I thought about my kids: a 24-year-old in college and a 12-year-old still living with me. *Don't panic? I could die here!*

Terrified, I wanted to cry. Determined to keep cool, I sat down and became aware of my breath. Deep breath. Inhale. Exhale.

My stomach cramped. My tongue swelled. My entire body was under attack.

"Where are they? Why are they taking so long? Are they almost here?" I asked every few minutes.

Twenty minutes later, the sound of the helicopter gave me hope. JP and two hikers waved their arms to help the pilot spot us. It's not easy to find little specks of people in a wide-open space from a helicopter.

A few minutes later, I was in the ER asking, "Doc, I'm going to be okay now, aren't I?"

"I don't know yet," he said.

It was not the answer I was looking for—the only time in my life I actually *wanted* a man to lie to me.

It wasn't long before complete sedation took away any fears. I was moved from the ER to intensive care. A large area around the bite turned black and blue. There was bluish discoloration under my nails. Muscles twitched. Doctors stated there was "severe envenomation."

"That first night was trying," JP later told me. "We figured if you got through the night, you'd make it. When I first saw you, there were three tubes down your throat and four people working on you. Your throat and tongue were very swollen."

"Critically ill in a life-threatening situation," stated my medical records. My mom had groups praying for me. JP sent out an email asking for prayers. I had my own little mantra: "Dear God, please make this nightmare end." I figured some good would come out of this. But while I waited for that silver lining, my leg was turning black! Temporarily paralyzed, I was helpless and dependent.

The venom attacked every system of my body, causing bruising and swelling from my toes to the top of my head. The texture of the skin on my abdomen, thighs, and groin became extremely stiff and painfully hard. It felt more like hard leather. I gained 60 pounds from swelling!

My side and ribs were bruised. The top of my foot blistered badly. I was anemic and had several blood transfusions. Seven days later, more antivenin. Who knew a snake could do so much damage?

"I was so scared when I saw you in the ICU. You were yellow," a friend later said.

During those two weeks, my son brought me a grand slam base-ball he'd hit and two other homerun balls! I told my nurse, "I'm going to need a trophy cabinet if they don't get me out of here pretty soon."

Fifteen days and at least 28 vials of antivenin later, I went home.

I had to learn to be more patient, as my physical healing was going to take time. I practiced gratitude more than ever—for everyone and everything. I became more compassionate.

Life can change in a split second. I could have died and never seen my kids again. The importance of always keeping peace with loved ones became very obvious after this ordeal.

I looked for something positive in my daily progress—first walking one house length, the next day two. Within a few weeks, I walked, albeit slowly, for a half hour. From the feeling I had inside, you'd have thought I ran a marathon.

My body healed. My leg has a couple of issues, but I am able to do anything and everything I want with that leg. I couldn't even move that leg for a few days. I had to learn how to walk again, but less than two years later I started training to get my fitness certifications and I now teach several Zumba® and senior fitness classes at various gyms.

Taking the first step is the start—then looking for the good all around—like the perfect day for a hike—with my new snake-proof boots!

So, patience and progress—a couple of the lessons learned. I was put in a position where I had no choice but to be patient. Healing would take time. I also learned dependence. There were a lot of people helping me in those first few weeks.

Believing we are all 100 percent responsible for everything in our lives, I had to ask myself: *So, how'd you bring this on? How did I attract this into my life?*

For one thing, here I was on a beautiful day hiking in nature, but my mind was busy taking a friend's inventory. In fact, I was doing exactly what I felt my friend was doing—thinking negatively.

"Was it a step backward?" I asked one of my spiritual teachers.

"It's not about the snake bite, it's about the experience and what comes from it," he said. "You never know if something's good or bad until God's done with it, and God's never done."

Our souls evolve. Based on our every experience, we grow and we make better choices—choices that are in alignment with the Divine.

From each better choice, Consciousness evolves. We are all encouraged and assisted by each other's growth. As we take a look back at times in our lives that were painful, times we might call negative, we can see how much we've grown and evolved.

CHAPTER 8

To Thine Own Self be True

AS MENTIONED, AFTER my world was turned upside down with my son's diagnosis of type 1 diabetes, I found a whole new way of looking at life in my search for healing and health. With this new knowledge, I was better able to deal with circumstances the following year. Acceptance and surrender may be a couple of the keys to happiness, but that doesn't mean there isn't heartbreak or grief. I shed tears and researched when my older child did what he needed to do in order to be the perfect expression of carrying out the motto: To thine own self be true.

What I Gained When I Lost My Daughter

(Originally published in *Chicken Soup for the Soul—The Magic of Mothers and Daughters*)

My little girl was a tomboy. Oftentimes strangers would refer to her as my son.

"Pierce her ears," my sisters advised.

I grew her hair out, too, but it didn't change anything. Rachael didn't seem bothered by the comments and, in fact, sometimes seemed to enjoy hearing someone call her a boy.

We lived in Hawaii when Rachael was in third and fourth grades. On May 1st, the kids participated in the Lei Day celebration with music and hula. The girls wore mu'umu'us and the boys aloha shirts. I have a photo from that day—she looked pained. That was the last time I made her wear a dress.

In hindsight, a friend said: "It might have been a good idea to just let her stay home that day."

When she was fifteen, we were living in San Diego. Rachael was excited about attending her first high school dance. When her date, Shawn, arrived, I took pictures of the two of them. As they got ready to leave, I kissed my daughter goodbye.

I'd already said everything that was on my mind—not the usual things parents tell their kids such as don't drink and drive. Instead, I told her to be cautious and aware, to watch her back, reminding her that some people are intolerant and ignorant.

I wanted the easiest possible lifestyle for my daughter. I didn't want to see her get hurt, harmed, threatened, antagonized, or taunted. Often that's what people resort to when they meet up with someone different from themselves.

I said a prayer, then called my sister. "Rachael just left for the dance. I did the normal mom things, taking pictures and all, but it was hard."

My sister listened patiently as I cried.

"Shawn looked beautiful in a gorgeous dress, her hair styled, her makeup perfect. Shawn's parents may have to deal with emotions similar to mine, but at least they got to see their daughter looking like a woman," I sniffled. "Rachael had her hair slicked back and was wearing a tux."

At nineteen, Rachael changed her name to Caoinlean Caleb, saying she wanted to choose her own name, something that had meaning to her.

Less than a year later, I received an email from my daughter. It was a short note but by the time I finished it, I was reading through a blur of tears.

"Hi Mom,

I need to tell you something and I thought it would be best to e-mail you so that you could process it before we talk. I know you've always said that you want your children to be happy, and there is one thing in particular that I need right now in order to be happy. You know I've always been a tomboy, but it is more than that. I was born into the wrong body, and I need to fix that now. I hope you can understand that. If you have questions about it, you can ask me. Love you."

Agony is the word that comes closest to describing how I felt in that moment. Tears flowed for a few seconds before the sound of pain escaped my throat.

The next few days were consumed with tears and heartache. I researched in an attempt to understand. I read that thirty percent of the transgender population commit suicide. At least my kid had the courage and strength to do what she felt was necessary to be true to herself—which could be keeping her alive. Or…should I say him?

It took a few days before I responded to the email from "my little girl."

"Dear Rachael,
I'm struggling right now and feeling a lot of pain. It's a grieving process; a loss. I do have many questions and in trying to understand I went online to do some research. I will wait with my questions until we talk. You know I love you no matter what. I hope you can understand how painful and difficult this is for a mother. We are not our bodies; we are our souls. Love, Mom

p.s. I don't need any more ideas for articles or books (just trying to keep a sense of humor here)."

We lived in different states and sometimes didn't see each other for several months, so I didn't realize she was already living as a guy—part of the process in order to obtain male hormones.

A few months after the email, s/he started taking male hormones and went to San Francisco to have chest surgery—removal of her large D-cup breasts. A large scar was left from surgery. Hair was growing on his chest. He had new nipples. He shaved his face instead of his legs.

In the interest of keeping things humorous, he gave me a greeting card for newborns, "Congratulations! It's a boy." It was a sweet card with him recognizing that I had a lot to deal with, too, in this decision he'd made. "Thanks for all of your support. I'm really proud of how you've been handling everything," he wrote.

It was a rough transition trying to remember he versus she, to see my former daughter now as a guy with a beard sitting at the breakfast table without a shirt on. It was difficult explaining things to my other child, who was seven at the time. His nickname for Rachael was "Sissy."

Sometimes I was in the middle of telling a story from years ago when he was a she and wondered: Do I refer to my son or my daughter? He was a she back then. An article on trans-etiquette cleared up that question—always refer to the person in the gender they are now. Also early on, I'd talk to someone and couldn't remember if they thought I had a daughter or a son. These things aren't covered in Parenting 101.

Questions would pop in my head and even if my new son thought they were weird, he was kind enough to reply.

"Is your sex drive now like that of an eighteen-year-old guy versus a twenty-year-old woman?"

"Yes."

"Did you take a sudden interest in sports after starting hormones?"

"No."

My younger son asked if Caleb is better at playing catch now.

Although heartbroken, I knew I had only one choice—acceptance. There were times when "hey, girl" slipped out of my mouth. It was a conscious effort to say he and him—but now it's become second nature.

I was clueless as to what my child was going through in high school. There was not a lot of information available at the time—even back in 2000 you didn't see transgender on informational programs.

On occasion I've pondered the question of whether I raised a daughter or a son. I guess it doesn't really matter. My child is a courageous, kind person that I'm proud to have as my kid, regardless of gender. The main thing is his happiness. My transgender child is the same person, with the same soul. I loved the daughter I lost and now I love the son I gained.

Now, 20 years later, my son is extremely happy with his life and who he is. What more could a mom ask for?

CHAPTER **9**

Laughter

FROM THE MOVIE *Anatomy of an Illness*, based on the book of the same name by Norman Cousins:

Norman asked his doctor, "If negative emotions can produce negative chemical changes, wouldn't positive ones produce positive chemical changes? Isn't it possible for love, hope, faith, laughter, confidence, the will to live, have therapeutic value?"

"Norman, there's nothing so revolutionary about that. All doctors know that a patient's attitude has a large bearing on healing," his doctor answered.

Norman then told his doctor that he wanted to change his treatment and added, "I want to start taking responsibility for myself."

His idea was to get off of painkillers and begin "massive doses" of vitamin C because that helps oxygenate the blood, which he figured might help with his joint inflammation.

Norman felt a hospital is not a place to get well. "The minute you fall asleep, someone will be in to change the sheets."

So Norman left the hospital, rented a room, and in addition to vitamin C, he used laughter in the form of funny movies to heal himself. He had been diagnosed with an autoimmune disease that was very painful and caused destruction in his joints. He found that after watching ten minutes of something funny that made him laugh, he could sleep pain-free for two hours. He eventually recovered from his illness.

His doctor told Norman he went along with Norman's plan "because you believed."

Norman went on to say, "Never underestimate the power of positive emotions nor the incredible regenerative powers of the mind and body."

Would this work for everyone? It's not just about the "healing method." It's about attitude and belief.

Humor is mankind's greatest blessing. ~ Mark Twain

Laughter affects your health—mentally, emotionally, and physically. It calms your nerves, reduces tension, and brightens your mood.

Research on the effects of laughter on the body shows it produces pain-killing endorphins. It decreases cortisol levels, which decreases stress. It strengthens the immune system, lowers blood pressure, decreases pain, helps reduce inflammation and tension in the body, and can even burn calories.

Driving to work? Think about a time something funny happened and laugh out loud. Like Cousins, you can watch movies and, nowadays, it's easy to find short, funny clips online. Reader's Digest knows the therapeutic value of a good laugh—they even named one of their columns, "Laughter, the Best Medicine."

To keep a good attitude, hang out with positive people.

You are the average of the five people you spend the most time with.
~ Jim Rohn

After a gathering with friends who uplift, inspire, and motivate, how do you think you're going to feel afterward versus a get-together with a bunch of negative Nellies? Positive people find it difficult to endure lunch with a crowd that's talking disease, drama, destruction, and "ain't it awful." In addition to being a downer, think of what you could have done with that time.

Attitude is everything. It's your entire outlook on the world and the people you meet. The key is to look for the good, even if you have to start small. Send someone light and love. Got a meeting with a boss you don't care for? Practice visualization and meditation beforehand.

When it comes to attitude, Dr. Bruce Lipton said in an interview that 90 percent of illness and disease is from stress. As for a healthy lifestyle, Lipton said it's about how you are responding to life. "It's not determined by your genes, but it's determined by your attitude about life."

I took a short course on aging. There was a question asking what's most important as we age. I was thinking the best response was community and camaraderie, which are very important, but the answer was attitude about aging.

People need people. The value of close friends, as well as a sense of community, is an important part of being happy and healthy. Some researchers say friends are more important than family for our health and happiness, especially as we age. One of the big reasons for this is that we can pick our friends. If a friendship no longer serves us, we can move on. For those that do make a difference in your life, spend time with them. Everyone gets busy, but it's important to make time for those who are important to you. Being a part of your community helps reduce stress and keeps your mental attitude up.

Hobbies are great for your attitude, and getting together with others who share similar interests is fun and enjoyable. These days it's so easy to find like-minded people. Meetup.com has groups with all kinds of different interests that meet regularly.

Speaking of friends, let's not forget the power of pets. Researchers at Miami University and Saint Louis University found that older people who own pets have fewer visits to the doctor than those without pets. Studies show an increased recovery in hospitalized, chronically ill patients and older patients when animal-assisted therapy and activities are used.

A friend of mine took her dog, Max, to juvenile halls, convalescent homes, and to visit people in hospice care. One woman they met had spent several months in a convalescent home, never talking to anyone, not one word, until she and Max stopped by one afternoon. As the woman petted Max, she began to tell my friend about the dog she had when she was a young girl. The staff at the home listened in amazement since they'd never heard that patient speak before. My friend said she witnessed numerous miracles but always felt she gained more than she gave.

Regardless of what you're doing, it seems that just having your dog present can make a difference in heart rate. Scientists attribute the therapeutic effects of pets to the non-judgmental, accepting nature of animals. Interaction with a pet is non-threatening and uncomplicated, which is not always the case with people. I remember as a teenager jokingly telling my dad that I thought he liked the dog better than us kids. "The dog doesn't talk back," he said, chuckling.

If you love animals but don't want the responsibility of owning a pet, there are plenty of places that appreciate volunteers—shelters, humane societies, and even neighbors needing a dog walker.

Volunteering is wonderful. It helps others, and most people who volunteer feel a sense of giving with their service. They may not realize it, but they're adding to the evolution of themselves, others, and the universe.

Smile more—even a fake smile contributes to well-being. Let go of the negative and replace it with the positive in order to create a positive, happy life.

CHAPTER 10

Meditation and Visualization

THE MOST IMPORTANT connection you can make is with God, the Universe, Consciousness. Meditation is a time for quieting the mind, going within, and connecting with Spirit. There are lots of books and videos on meditation, as well as guided meditations to listen to that will help you relax into a calm state of mind so that you're better able to quiet your thoughts. Breathing exercises are great. If your mind wants to chatter, give gratitude, and bring your focus back to your breath. Taking just a few minutes to meditate each morning can make a difference with a more positive vibration and how you respond to life's happenings throughout your day. You're not alone when it comes to mind chatter. Just keep coming back to the breath and do your best to stay focused.

Visualization is a way of creating what you'd like to bring into your world. Your possibilities are limitless, so let your imagination go wild. Vividly see the picture playing out in your mind and feel how you would feel when your vision becomes your reality. What you feel, you attract.

Ask yourself questions. If you want to earn more money, how much? When you charge what you're worth, how do you feel? What would make you feel successful? If you had (fill in the blank), what would it look like right now? What would change in your life? Tune yourself to be in harmony with the outcome you want and expect it. Vibrate thoughts and feelings to accompany your visualization. If it's a job, give out the feelings, "I got the job! I am so happy and grateful!" In your imagination, see the office, feel yourself shaking a new colleague's hand. Who are you going to share your good news with? Picture them, too, as you excitedly tell them.

Now go back and do it again. If your mind wanders, bring it back to the outcome. See the results you want. Feel the joy. Feel the gratitude as you give thanks.

A study at the University of Chicago showed the power of visualization involving free throws. Several students were selected randomly and split into three groups. They tested to see how many shots each group could make from the free throw line. Then, for 30 days, the first group did nothing. The second group practiced free throws for an hour a day. The third group visualized making free throws for an hour every day. After 30 days, the first group kept the same percentage, not getting better or worse. The second group improved by 24 percent. The third group using visualization improved by 23 percent—without even touching a basketball.

Visualization Exercise

Close your eyes. Quiet the mind. If you have trouble with that, listen to a guided meditation or practice something like the Silva Method™, which is available as a book or seminar. You don't have to hold your new picture for very long—try just 30 seconds or so. Are you seeing health instead of illness, success instead of failure? Get into the feeling place you'd be in as if you'd already achieved what you desire.

Capture the feeling associated with your realized wish by assuming the feeling that would be yours were you already in possession of the thing you desire, and your wish will objectify itself.
~ Neville Goddard

Relaxation Exercise – Progressive Relaxation

Progressive relaxation is tightening a muscle group as you inhale, hold for five seconds or so, then relaxing the muscles as you exhale. I work the muscles in a certain order from head to toe, but if you prefer, do it bottom to top. Hold each group for five seconds.

1. Tighten the facial muscles. Hold for five seconds. Exhale.
2. Lift the shoulders toward the ears. Hold and exhale.
3. Tighten the arms and make fists. Hold and exhale.
4. Tighten the abs. Hold and exhale.
5. Tighten the legs and butt. Hold and exhale.
6. Curl the toes. Hold and exhale.

Breathe in; breathe out. Vibrate and resonate with the abundance of life. If need be, get rid of any memory of lack. Fill yourself with peace. Go deeper into a calm, relaxed state. See things the way you want them to be. Image the outcome.

Keep the faith. Keep your connection to Source Energy and your vision. Focus on beautiful, harmonious thoughts. Be open to receive.

"I accept all the generous gifts that life has for me now."

"Everything I have prospers."

Infinite Intelligence is guiding you in all ways. You choose your images, thoughts, and feelings that are controlling your destiny.

Everything in life, including happiness and unhappiness, is a state of mind. What you believe and feel to be true will come to pass. Thoughts are things, and you have the power to change your thoughts.

Keep practicing. Make a commitment to practice visualization for at least a few minutes every day for at least thirty days. Successful musicians and athletes practice, practice, practice. Doubts and negative thoughts are nothing more than habits. Get rid of doubt—it screws up images.

Nature is a great pick-me-up. Consider all the meditation music interspersed with sounds of nature—oceans, rivers, birds, and lots of others. Sunlight can affect your mood, too.

Getting in touch with Mother Earth is grounding and can give an attitude adjustment: gardening, walking barefoot in the grass or on a sandy beach, even pulling weeds.

If you don't know for sure what you want or are in a state of confusion, pray. Go within and ask a question, then listen for an answer. When I was in my early twenties, I was offered a job at a brand-new radio station. It sounded like an exciting, fun adventure. But I had just relocated and started a new job a few months earlier. The new job would require another relocation. I did visit the new station but thought it would be best to stay put. I prayed, though, asking for guidance. Not only that, but I also specifically asked God to make it obvious. I didn't want to be wondering what some "sign" meant. Shortly thereafter, I was fired. Ouch! For no good reason. And that was the only time that ever happened in my career. An hour later I was on the phone and had the job I'd been contemplating. I moved that weekend. It turned out to be a great choice. Now, though, I do preface my prayers with "I'd like an answer, but I don't want to get hurt."

A few months later I got a call from the station that canned me, asking me to come back. The manager had been let go, and the new one wanted me back. I turned the job down, but it was nice to get the offer.

CHAPTER 11

Words are Powerful

THE UNIVERSE TAKES our words literally, even if that's not what we mean and not what we want to create.

Example: "I can't stand..." You hear people say that one fairly often. The Universe is always listening, and you don't want to end up on crutches or in a wheelchair—no longer able to stand. A friend of mine used that expression frequently. I reminded her to watch her words.

Then one day while she was hiking, she broke her arm. As a dental assistant, she was unable to work.

I said to her, "I thought you would break a leg or something where you wouldn't be able to stand since you were always saying, 'I can't stand.'"

"If that had happened, I'd still be able to work, standing. But I can't work without my arm, so I'm home sitting around," she replied.

When your conscious mind puts out messages, the subconscious mind does whatever it's instructed to do, without question and without analyzing whether something is good for you or not.

In this creative process, whatever direction you, the Soul, give to Spirit, Spirit will create for you.

The outcome and results are your life: your body, your environment, and everything that's happening. They are the effects. Since the law of cause and effect is always in operation, it's up to you to figure out the cause if you want to change the effect.

What are you saying to yourself and others? Are you complaining about your job, your circumstances, your partner, your family? Sometimes we feel the need to vent, but then it's time to move on.

If you're in an undesirable situation, you may need to confide in someone and get guidance to help you figure out what to do. But to keep focusing on the situation and badmouthing it does not help. It only makes it worse because that's where you're putting your attention.

One of my jobs during my broadcast career was reporting from a news helicopter. I'd been at that job for almost 20 years. I was over it and ready for something new, but I stayed on. One of the pilots I worked with, who'd only been flying with the company for a year, often complained about his frustration with the job. Probably not a good idea for the two of us to be flying together with those thoughts and words. One afternoon after covering a story, we headed back to our base and as we went to land, we crashed. Neither one of us went back to that job, and fortunately, we're both okay. Here's the scoop...

Crash Landing

The summer of 2019 is forever burned in my brain, literally, and I am so grateful it was not my last. The heat and stickiness of one August afternoon felt even more so, cramped in our small space 1,000 feet above San Diego. As a reporter and photographer in the only television news helicopter in our county, I shot footage for several stations. When my pilot and I got a call to launch to a breaking news story near the coast, we looked forward to temperatures being a little cooler. A small brush fire had turned into a larger spectacle. The flames spread to a nearby auto dealership with several vehicles burning.

After orbiting the scene and reporting the details, we flew back to our base. Near the hangar, we had a platform we land on called a dolly. We were about to touch down when, without warning, the chopper missed the dolly and smashed to the ground with a thunderous bang. It flipped over on its top, and as the rotor blades struck the ground, the helicopter came to a screeching halt on its side. It happened in an instant. Terrified of what could happen next, I was overcome with a feeling that I wasn't ready to die.

My pilot turned around with a look on his face that I'd never seen before and never want to see again. There was an urgency in his voice, his eyes intense.

Stunned, I looked around, taking in the scene. So much equipment, the camera laptop, two-way radios, phones, shattered windows—everything was scattered. As if in slow motion, I saw his mouth move.

"Are you okay?" he asked. I realized I could hear him. He didn't have his headset on. Neither did I. They were thrown off our heads during the crash. All was eerily quiet. The helicopter's engine was no longer running.

It was at that moment that panic set in with an overwhelming sensation of dread. My mind sprinted from thought to thought. *Is this it? Am I going to die right now?* And then the scariest thought of all... *was this whole thing about to go up in flames?* My breath caught in my throat. *Was this the moment before I died?*

My entire being wanted out of that helicopter. I think my mouth was saying words, but I can't be sure. My eyes darted from the door to the window to the other door to the seat belt that still held me tightly. All of my weight was heaved to one side making the seat belt taut. *How do I get out of this?*

"Get me out of here," I started to repeat incessantly. "Get me out of this helicopter."

I felt throbbing inside my head.

Then suddenly a miracle happened. The door to the helicopter opened. My soon-to-be hero's arm reached inside.

"My seat belt," I said. My stomach was tied in knots. I felt stuck. In one swift motion, the man undid my seat belt, grabbed my hands, picked me up, and pulled me out of the helicopter, placing me safely on the ground.

"Are you okay?" he asked.

"No," I repeated over and over. "No."

Shocked, I stood frozen with wide eyes as the man went back to help the pilot.

Smoke started pouring from the back of the helicopter. More people surrounded us. I felt a mixture of panic and relief. Someone jolted me out of my daze. He grabbed my hand and yanked me, running toward the hangar. When we stopped, I turned and looked back. Smoke, dirt, and debris were strewn everywhere. The tail rotor broke off and the main rotor blades crumbled.

Taking all of this in, I said, "I need a hug." His big bear hug gave me comfort.

Sirens blared as an ambulance and fire trucks arrived.

Paramedics escorted me inside. They bandaged three of my toes that were painful and bleeding. I have no idea what cut them.

"They hurt really bad," I said. "My head, too."

"With a head injury, it's best to get it checked out," they said.

The helicopter was leaking fuel with my phone trapped in it. I thought I knew my son's number, so once in the ambulance, the paramedic tried calling him. Wrong number.

The ER doctor stitched my toes, and a CAT scan showed no bleeding in my head.

One of the nurses found my records in their files and there were a couple of contact numbers listed. She called one of them. "Your friend is on his way to pick you up," she said.

When I caught up with my son a half-hour later, I hugged him tightly. Tears rolled down my cheeks. "I haven't had a chance to cry," I said.

I could see the relief in his eyes, but his face showed concern. He wondered, he said, if there'd be any long-term effects on my mind and body.

He drove me to the airport so I could get my car.

My pilot handed me my phone like a package wrapped in a tissue with a strong stench of fuel.

"You're going to be sore tomorrow. You were just in a helicopter crash. Leave your car and let your son drive you home."

"I need my car," I said. "I teach a class at the YMCA tomorrow morning."

"Forget about the class."

My son and I left the building.

"I'm driving my car," I said.

By the time I got home, the "troubled landing" had become a news story. I had tons of voice and text messages:

"Are you ok?? I just saw the chopper crashed!!!!"

"Just got a text about the chopper. I'm freaking out here."

"Jo, as soon as you're able, PLEASE text me. I've been praying for you."

Although my phone was covered in fuel, I managed to let close friends and family know I was okay before attempting sleep.

My head pounded and I was tired, but instead of sleep, I tossed and turned as I kept replaying the afternoon over and over. I tried to clear my thoughts and meditate, but my mind immediately returned to the crash.

I had instructions to keep my toes covered, so the next morning, I put on my tennis shoes and headed for the Y. I'm not sure what I was thinking; perhaps I was still in a state of shock because for the next hour, I taught a fitness class. I walked the dog, too, and within a few days, my toes became irritated and inflamed, requiring antibiotics. Our bodies can heal, but it's important to take responsibility and do our part, such as take it easy when needed.

I took a break from flying, but after several months, I still felt anxious at the thought of getting back in a helicopter. I sought counseling and eventually decided not to continue flying. I returned to work reporting from the ground.

The crash shook me up, but I felt blessed to be alive and well. Thank goodness because the day before I had a colonoscopy. Imagine that for an exciting last day on earth. The helicopter incident was a reminder that we never really know what the next moment will bring. While I do believe everything happens for a reason, I also think we are creators. Maybe this was a wake-up call to make a change. I'd been working airborne for close to two decades and for quite some time was ready for something different. My pilot often said he was no longer enjoying the job. The crash motivated both of us to move forward. For me, that meant slowing down and spending more quality time with my family, and nurturing friendships.

I came to realize it's okay to not always get back on the horse. Maybe the braver thing is to leave the horse behind and tame a new challenge altogether.

Focus and Intention

Put your attention on what you want. If people want to steer you into a conversation that is not healthy, don't get sucked in. When you understand this and the impact it will have on your health, you'll take note and use discipline to make sure you are emitting words that will bring about what you desire. You are the creator of your world.

When you engage in fearful conversation, your attention is going to what scares you and what you don't want. Changing that to a hopeful exchange will completely change the vibration. You can't put your attention on both the positive and the negative at the same time, but you can replace one with the other.

Sharing your health experiences with others needing help and compassion is a way to contribute to your community. It can be done in a positive way by looking for the good. Instead of discussing chemo or radiation, tell others about the wonderful growth spurts that came into your world that you would not have experienced otherwise. How did you evolve from this? That's putting your focus on the positive aspect of some of the trials and tribulations you experience. It might not happen right away, and while it can be therapeutic to talk about our struggles, in order to move forward, we eventually need to start talking about what has been gained from the experience.

Talking about what you *want* is more fun and brings more blessings into your life.

In my own experience, my spiritual growth and the knowledge I gained after my son was diagnosed with type 1 diabetes were phenomenal.

Experiments have been done to show the power of intention. This is from an article entitled "Can group meditation prevent violent crime? Surprisingly, the data suggests yes" on EurekAlert.org: "Large groups practicing the advanced Transcendental Meditation program were associated with significant reductions in U.S. homicide and urban violent crime rates during an intervention period of 2007-2010." Many would not find that surprising, knowing the power of intention.

It's important to keep your intentions for yourself and your loved ones positive and loving. What happens is that we often create unconsciously. Since our mind has the ability to turn what we're focused on into reality, it's important to do so consciously. Challenge yourself to become more and more aware of what you're focusing on.

Gossiping is an extremely negative form of talk. It will stunt your spiritual growth. If you want to evolve and better yourself, knock off the gossip. While this includes what you say, it also includes what's going into your ears and mind. If you're listening to someone else gossip, you're a part of it.

> *Great minds discuss ideas; average minds discuss events;*
> *small minds discuss people.*
> *~ Eleanor Roosevelt*

Gossip is a very popular pastime. Standing in line at the grocery store, we are bombarded with magazines filled with what's happening in the lives of celebrities. Whatever happened to *Time* and *Newsweek* at the front counter?

Watch your words. They are powerful.

Someone told me a story of a woman who became ill and was hospitalized. After doing some tests, the doctor told the woman's husband that his wife had a terminal illness and didn't have much longer to live. The man told the doctor not to say a word to his wife. (This was several decades ago). He went to his wife's room, told her she had the flu, and took her home. She lived for many more years. Had she been given a terminally ill diagnosis, things could have turned out quite differently. Not knowing it, she didn't dwell on it and it wasn't a part of her belief.

I was listening to a recording from Deepak Chopra where he told the story of a medical doctor who decided to get a life insurance plan. One of the requirements was a physical examination. A large, dark spot was found on one of his lungs, and he was told he had inoperable cancer. The man died a few months later.

Deepak later discovered an old x-ray of the man from 25 years earlier. It had that same dark spot on the lung. Belief is a strong force.

Are you listening to fearful words from the media, religion, or the government? If it makes you fearful or gives you feelings of scarcity, turn it off. Then replace those words in your mind to faith and hope. Expect everything to work out.

As people became fearful during the pandemic, a friend and spiritual teacher said to me: "As one grows in faith, the illnesses of fear are replaced by health. No laboratory, no doctor, nothing can compete with the Innate Intelligence already built within you."

Even simple things like "Don't forget" can be replaced with "Remember."

We hear the expression "caught" a cold. Throw it back. How about this: Maybe instead of "catching a cold," you're stressed or worried, so your immune system is down and you're unable to resist germs that then manifest as a cold. Maybe the worry can be attributed to the fear you felt when you heard how awful everything is. We are creators.

Knowing how powerful you are doesn't mean you'll never create something like ill health. We are works in progress, disciplining ourselves to become more aware and conscious. There are still times when we act unconsciously. With knowledge, we learn to figure out the cause.

Like thoughts, keep your speech directed toward what you want, not what you don't want.

Spirit simply takes your words and thoughts and carries out your orders. What are you ordering?

CHAPTER 12

You Gotta Love Your Body

You are what you eat, so don't be fast, cheap, easy, or fake.
~ Unknown

Fuel Your Vehicle

IF YOU DON'T maintain your car, it'll eventually break down. The same is true of your body. Why put junk into your body if you want it to keep on running?

The body is your temple. Treat it right and with respect. Your body is an effect, not a cause. If you let that soak in, it means that every ailment, an effect, has a cause. We create our bodies. Fueling it with junk food and sitting on the couch all day will have an effect. When dis-ease "happens," start asking yourself questions. How was this caused? In addition to food and movement, think about your words, thoughts, and actions. Have you been stressed out, which is all too often the cause of illness? What might have brought on this bout of the flu or cold? No one consciously asks for these things. That's why it helps to get present and get off autopilot. Recognizing the cause and taking responsibility gives you the freedom and power to heal it. Notice how your positive changes and choices help you achieve a healthier body.

Eating healthy can be time consuming and it requires a commitment. You're worth it. It might be a lot quicker to drive through a fast-food restaurant than it is to cut up fruits and vegetables, although I have seen people wait in very long lines at a drive-through in order to get take-out. It's a lifestyle change. Life gets busy, so do your prep. Here are some tips:

- When you have time off, do your grocery shopping and try new, healthy recipes.
- Prepare for the week by chopping fruits and vegetables on the weekend and making dishes to take to work. There's also the alternative of buying your produce already chopped, but it does cost a little more.
- Don't wait until you're famished to eat. In case that does happen, preparing healthy snacks ahead of time is helpful. Veggies and hummus or a handful of nuts are a good way to curb the appetite.
- Give up the high-calorie fast food. Cut down on going out for meals. When you do go out, choose restaurants that offer healthy options. Many portions are large—split the meal with someone or get half of it to go.
- Download an app such as CalorieKing: https://www.calorieking.com/us/en/. It gives you the lowdown on calories, carbs, fat, cholesterol, sodium, and protein. It has food categories, food brands, and fast-food chains. Or ask the server for the nutritional menu. It's surprising the number of calories in some of those salads on the menu. Most restaurant dishes are higher in fat, carbs, and calories than the healthy choices you can make at home.

This doesn't mean you'll never eat your favorite food again. Have a day to treat yourself. Check out cookbooks from the library and try new healthy recipes. Keep in mind, though, that some cookbooks that are touted as healthy might not be. Some of them call for a lot of processed foods—yep, another thing to eliminate. In time, you'll find recipes that are nutritious, delicious treats, like dips and raw veggies.

Buy Organic

The body is constantly rebuilding, using the nutrients, vitamins, and minerals from the foods you eat. Pesticides can affect your health. Sometimes, though, your pocketbook may tell you to scrub and clean those non-organic cucumbers twice as hard. The Environmental Working Group (EWG) compiled a list of fruits and vegetables with the highest level of pesticide residues. They call it the "Dirty Dozen." The group also puts together the "Clean Fifteen," a list of fruits and veggies with the fewest concentrations of pesticides. These lists change annually.

Dirty Dozen:

1. Strawberries
2. Spinach
3. Kale/collard/mustard greens
4. Nectarines
5. Apples
6. Grapes
7. Cherries
8. Peaches
9. Pears
10. Bell and hot peppers
11. Celery
12. Tomatoes

Clean 15:

1. Avocados
2. Sweet Corn
3. Pineapples
4. Onions
5. Papayas
6. Frozen sweet peas
7. Eggplant

8. Asparagus
9. Broccoli
10. Cabbage
11. Kiwifruit
12. Cauliflower
13. Mushrooms
14. Honeydew
15. Cantaloupe

Cleansing from the Inside Out

You can tell if you're clean from the inside out by looking at your skin. Skin is the last place to get nutrition, so if your skin is clear and radiant, so are your insides.

A great way to start your day is with a cleansing drink—a smoothie or juice. Here are a few suggestions of foods to keep you clean and healthy:

- Aloe vera—this plant is a beauty product and healing agent. It is commonly used as a treatment for burns, including sunburn. Aloe vera has all kinds of great benefits. Cut sections from a larger plant or pick up a bottle of aloe vera juice and add a little to your smoothie.
- Parsley—curly or Italian, this herb has way more benefits than just sitting pretty on your plate. It cleans your blood supply, is great for fresh breath, and is loaded with nutrients. Put a handful or more in your smoothie or juice.
- Cilantro—may possibly bind with and remove heavy metals such as mercury and is a powerful cleanser.
- Chia seeds—absorb bile salts released by the liver; high in omega-3 fatty acids; rich in antioxidants; provides fiber, calcium, and iron.

Top off your smoothie with some greens like spinach or kale, along with a scoop of green powder, and a little bit of frozen fruit, and take on the day.

Balance Your pH Level

A pH scale runs from 1 to 14 with 7 being neutral and 7.4 a good balance for your body. Eating the proper balance of alkaline and acidic foods will help you achieve that balance. You can purchase pH strips to test yourself.

The cells become more fertile for diseases to develop when the body is acidic. A few other effects include allergies, fatigue, headaches, joint and muscle pain, ulcers, and inflammation. What you eat and drink has an effect on the pH level of your body, but even more important are your thoughts. Negative emotions and thoughts such as worry and anger are acidic, too.

You can find lists of alkaline and acidic foods online. Here are just a few:

Acidic—sugar, processed foods, and soft drinks.

Alkaline—almonds, endive, garlic, ginger, spinach, lentils, sweet potatoes, cucumbers, millet, most fresh veggies, and some fruits such as avocado and coconut.

Tidbit on Protein

How much? If you're pumping lots of iron you might need to up your intake of protein, but according to *Eat, Drink, and Be Healthy* by Walter C. Willett, M.D., the recommended daily allowance for protein is just over 7 grams per 20 pounds of body weight. That comes out to about 50 grams for a 140-pound person; close to 65 grams for a 180-pound person. Lots of foods contain protein. People on vegan diets don't typically lack protein; it's B-12 that might be low.

If you choose meat as your source of protein, it's best to go organic and free range. Organic means the animal received no hormones, antibiotics, or human-made pesticides in its feed, which could include corn and/or soy. A grass-fed animal was pasture-raised and was not fed corn or soy.

How much is a hamburger worth? Willett mentions "The Consumer's Guide to Effective Environmental Choices" report stating that meat consumption "is the second most environmentally costly consumer activity. It takes 20 pounds of feed, usually corn, to make one pound of edible beef." This is not referring to a grass-fed animal. Also, corn is one of the most common genetically modified foods.

Tony Robbins concurs, "If Americans reduced their meat consumption by 10 percent, we would free 12 million tons of grain annually for human consumption, which would feed the entire 60 million who starve to death each year."

Consider occasional alternatives for protein. All kinds of nuts and beans are great sources of protein. Lots of vegetables are, too—a cup of broccoli has three grams of protein, a cup of spinach has one gram, and kale has over four grams per cup.

Calcium—Food for Thought

Eye-opener: According to *The China Study* by T. Colin Campbell and Thomas M. Campbell:

> Countries that use the most cow's milk and its products also have the highest fracture rates and the worst bone health [...] Researchers (at Yale University School of Medicine) explained that animal protein, unlike plant protein, increases the acid load in the body. An increased acid load means that our blood and tissues become more acidic. The body does not like this acidic environment and begins to fight it. In order to neutralize the acid, the body uses calcium, which acts as a very effective base. This calcium, however, must come from somewhere. It ends up being pulled from the bones, and the calcium loss weakens them, putting them at a great risk for fracture.

Willett (*Eat, Drink and be Healthy*) talks about several studies showing "that the more protein consumed, the more calcium excreted in the urine. When it comes to leaching calcium from bone, animal protein is somewhat more powerful than vegetable protein." Higher protein consumption is known to increase urinary calcium excretion.

Campbell, on his website nutritionalstudies.org, agrees:

High-protein diets – especially protein of animal foods – can cause the body to excrete more calcium than it gets. For example, a person eating 142 grams of protein a day – which some Americans do – will excrete twice as much calcium in the urine as a person taking in a more moderate 47 grams. Because our bodies need calcium to regulate many different activities, such as the functioning of our muscles and nerves, the deficit caused by too much protein causes the body to withdraw more calcium from our main calcium reserve "banks" – our bones, which become increasingly more fragile as calcium is removed from them.

I'll Drink to That!

Your body is 50 to 75 percent water—your brain is 95 percent water, blood 92 percent water, and lungs close to 90 percent. With numbers like that, water is a key ingredient to health, cleansing and flushing the body, carrying nutrients to the cells, and keeping your body functioning—your heart, your brain, your muscles, getting rid of bacteria from your bladder, and helping to keep you regular in the bathroom.

Feeling a little sleepy in the middle of the day? Mild dehydration can make you feel tired, especially after exercise. Instead of a nap, maybe all you need is a glass of water. Fluids from water, as well as foods such as fruits and vegetables, help your body replenish water that is lost.

You might need a little more H_2O if you have any of the following:

- Muscle cramps
- Low blood pressure

- Dizziness or confusion
- Tired/sleepy/lack of concentration
- Decreased urination
- Headache
- Dry skin

Something as simple as staying hydrated can do so much:

- Help repair joints and cartilage
- Aid in weight loss
- Put you in a better mood
- Strengthen teeth and bones
- Improve memory and proper functioning of the brain
- Reduce the risk of disease
- Energize you; add a little lemon to your water or try coconut water after a workout

Close to 30 percent of American adults have high blood pressure. When your blood is hydrated, it moves with ease down the freeways of your arteries and veins. Hydration makes your heart's job easier.

Our organs need lots of water to do their jobs. Without enough water, organs, along with every cell and system of our body, have to work harder, causing us to age faster. Want to slow the aging process and look and feel younger? Drink water. So simple, so easy. The list goes on, but you get the idea.

Preferably, use purified, filtered water. Perk it up with slices of cucumber, mint, orange, lemon—whatever sounds good to you.

What about Fats?

Fats provide your body energy, support cell growth, and protect and cushion your organs. They also assist in absorbing and transporting some nutrients to cells. Not all fats are bad for you, and you do need a certain amount for a healthy, balanced diet. Consideration needs to be given to good versus saturated fats. Unsaturated fats typically come from plant sources. They're liquid at room temperature and help reduce the risk of heart disease, lower cholesterol levels, and ease inflammation, as well as other benefits. The two main types of unsaturated fats are polyunsaturated/monounsaturated fats.

Food with polyunsaturated fats include walnuts, which contain omega-3 fatty acids, helping lower triglycerides and LDL cholesterol. Fish oil has omega-3 fats, and oils such as soybean and safflower contain omega-6 fats. Some of the foods containing monosaturated fats include cashews, almonds, and avocados.

The American Heart Association recommends limiting your intake of saturated fats. Saturated fats are found largely in animal foods, such as meat, whole milk, cheese, and butter, to name a few.

Trans fats are solid at room temperature and are best to avoid and preferably eliminate from your diet. Many processed and pre-packaged foods are high in trans fats, which are formed using what's called hydrogenation, a process when a liquid is transformed into a solid form. It preserves food for a longer time. They raise your low-density cholesterol levels, sometimes referred to as bad cholesterol, and lower good high-density cholesterol levels. Trans fats can increase your risk of developing heart disease and stroke. Check labels, but some of the foods you may find with trans fat include cakes, cookies, biscuits, fried fast foods, non-dairy creamers, whipped topping, and doughnuts.

Not All Carbs are Created Equal

Our bodies use carbohydrates for fuel. There are different types of carbs, though—simple and complex. Both turn to glucose in the body and give us energy.

Simple carbohydrates are sugars and come under lots of different names—glucose, dextrose, fructose, galactose. They're typically found in processed foods that lack nutrients: soda, juice, cookies, candy, white flour, white pasta, white rice, and white bread. Instead, choose brown rice and whole wheat pasta. Try spaghetti squash or Shirataki miracle noodles. They're made with Konjac flour, which contain prebiotics, have very few calories or carbohydrates, and improve digestion. Complex carbs are just that. They're unprocessed foods with vitamins, minerals, and fiber: peas, beans, whole grains, fruit, vegetables, nuts, seeds, and legumes.

Fruits are good for you. They're natural. They're plants. And although they contain sugar, they're also full of fiber, vitamins, minerals, and antioxidants. The fiber slows down the absorption of the sugar.

Glycemic Index

In a nutshell, glycemic index (GI) is a number given to a carbohydrate and has to do with how quickly the blood sugar elevates after eating a particular food. Certain foods raise your blood glucose level quickly (high GI), while others take their time (low GI). You won't get those blood sugar spikes followed by crashes when you eat whole foods that are loaded with nutrients and fiber. Stick with the complex carbs.

These are just a few ideas to help fuel your body and keep it healthy and energized. Even if you make one slight change in a positive direction, that's a good thing.

Get Rid of Toxins—In Your Home and In Your Body

Many people are worried about getting sick from germs. Take a look at the household products you use to sanitize your home. Many of them contain toxins that can be more harmful than germs. Consider buying all-natural, organic, and fragrance-free products or making your own. There's a lot you can do with baking soda, white vinegar, and essential oils.

Check the ingredients in products you buy—from cleaning supplies to perfumes. If you see the word "fragrance" included, there's a good chance it contains phthalates, which have been shown to disrupt hormones and cause obesity, birth defects, early puberty in girls, and low sperm count and insulin resistance in men. Children are particularly susceptible due to their continually changing hormone levels. Exposure to phthalates is usually from inhalation, but it can also occur through contact with your skin, such as washing your hands with certain soaps.

Some cleaning agents such as glass cleaner and polishes may have ammonia, which is hard on the lungs and, if used often, could lead to asthma or bronchitis. Carpet and upholstery cleaning solutions and dry-cleaning products could contain perchloroethylene (perc). The health hazards associated with perchloroethylene prompted the Environmental Protection Agency to ban the use of perc in residential buildings by 2020 and the state of California to eliminate it entirely by 2023.

Tips for a healthier home

- Instead of dry cleaning, try professional "wet cleaning" that avoids chemical solvents.
- Tea tree oil is antifungal. Try a few drops mixed with a little vinegar. Put in a spray bottle with water and you've got a safe, natural, all-purpose cleaner that kills germs. Lemon and eucalyptus essential oils are also great for all-purpose cleaners.
- Add a few drops of lemon to your cleaning sponge to help clean bacteria and germs from your kitchen counter.
- Peppermint essential oil with water in a spray bottle makes a safe, natural pesticide around the house. For ants or mice, put a few drops of peppermint oil on a cotton ball and leave it in areas where these pests are hanging out.
- Freshen the air with a few drops of essential oils in a diffuser. If you don't have a diffuser, put boiling water in a bowl and add the scent of your choice.
- In place of a dryer sheet, put a few drops of essential oil on a damp washcloth and throw it in the dryer with your clothes.

Tips for a healthier body

Pay attention to your body. It lets you know when you're not doing well—stomach aches, muscle tension, headaches, rising heart rate, clenched jaw or hands—are all signs your body is struggling.

Something as simple as a thought can produce stress in your body. Transforming thoughts from negative to positive is important because our inner world creates our outer world. Stress, worry, and anxiety can interfere with appetite, sleep, and relationships, and cause all kinds of health problems including substance abuse and other addictive behaviors.

According to the Mayo Clinic's website, "stress that's left unchecked can contribute to many health problems, such as high blood pressure, heart disease, obesity and diabetes." The site listed some of the common effects of stress:

- Sleeping problems
- Muscle tension or pain
- Fatigue
- Irritability
- Upset stomach
- Change in sex drive
- Chest pain

Headaches, heart disease, obesity, depression, sexual dysfunction, autoimmune diseases, and dilated blood vessels are other issues linked to long-term stress.

Anger and fear are feelings that bring on similar reactions to the body as stress. Your muscles tense, even spreading to the sympathetic nervous system, which is responsible for triggering the fight or flight response, causing circulatory changes.

Getting rid of germs in your environment by using natural products helps eliminate toxins. But stress and worry bring on more illness and disease than any germs. Consider what I call "mind gel"—something to rid the mind of negative thoughts and emotions.

Knowing all the harmful effects of a toxic mind, you can see how important it is to pay attention to your thoughts. It takes practice and it doesn't happen overnight, but with practice comes improvement.

CHAPTER 13

Keep Your Vehicle Tuned-Up

We do not stop exercising because we grow old—
we grow old because we stop exercising.
~Dr. Kenneth Cooper, Fitness Pioneer and "Father of Aerobics"

WHO LOOKS BACK at you when you look in the mirror? Is it a vibrant person, reflecting the energy you feel inside? Or is it someone you don't recognize—who looks tired and pale, maybe even unhealthy? When you're feeling fatigued or exhausted, exercise might be the last thing on your mind. Studies have shown, though, that regular exercise can increase feelings of energy. Researchers at the University of Georgia found that a low-intensity workout, such as a leisurely walk, increased energy levels more than a more intense workout. It helps recharge your batteries, and it doesn't have to be hard or expensive—even if you only do a few minutes. One four-letter word is the key—move.

Nutrition plays a major role in the health of your body, but your body has to absorb and distribute those nutrients. Exercising helps keep your digestive tract healthy and pushes food through it for better absorption. Our joints and muscles need to move, and when they do, they distribute nutrients to all parts of the body. Physical activity keeps you healthy, both physically and mentally. If you're feeling pain such as a sore back, stiff legs, or hip pain, the reason could be lack of exercise. Like drugs, alcohol, and smoking, inactivity is a health risk. Moving your body stimulates various brain chemicals resulting in a happier, more relaxed state.

Body movement increases your metabolism, improves circulation, strength, and stamina, gives you energy, keeps you toned, strengthens bones and the heart, gets the heart rate up—and keeps it up. Even after exercise, your metabolism stays higher.

Exercise really is a cure-all. High blood pressure? Exercise. Achy joints? Get moving! Need to lose weight? Exercise. It's for your health. Stressed out? Head for the gym. Feeling down? Get those endorphins going. You'll feel better and stronger, improve your attitude, and, as a nice bonus, you'll look better.

Let's Get Moving

There are so many fun ways to get moving. Take your choice and find something you enjoy. Biking, jogging, and dancing—with or without a partner. Walking, skiing, swimming, and hiking. The outdoors is a great place to be active. Hiking is a wonderful way to enjoy nature and keep fit. Even after my encounter with a rattle-snake (see Chapter 7), I still hike, typically only in the winter and with snakeproof boots. Find your favorite trails or explore new ones. There are books and apps on the market that give a rundown of all kinds of hiking trails, the distance, how long the hike will take, the best time of year, and the degree of difficulty.

For the stay-at-home athlete, there are plenty of ways to keep fit. Exercise machines are great for those who have the room and funds or keep it simple and low-cost with a large exercise ball, rebounder, resistance bands, or jump rope. To help with motivation and discipline, check out exercise videos online.

Joining a gym brings a new realm of possibilities and motivation: stationary bikes, treadmills, elliptical machines, stair steppers, rowing machines, and weights, as well as exercise classes where you can make new friends. There are plenty of classes for all ages and different degrees of intensity: cycling, various types of yoga, boot camps, boxing, aerobic step, Zumba®, strength and conditioning, and water aerobics.

If you're in a class that's a little too intense for you, modify it to your level. Trainers are also available at most clubs to help you learn how to use the strength and cardiovascular machines. You can mix it up with a class one day and machines the next—whatever works for you. Another advantage to a gym is that you can exercise regardless of the weather. If you're feeling a little hesitant or intimidated about joining a gym or going to a class, find a friend to go with you. You can be accountability partners, too.

If you're just getting started, especially if it's been a while since you've been active with an exercise program, talk with your doctor first. Start slowly and work your way up. Do what you can and be proud of yourself every step of the way. It's all about having fun and staying fit—for you and your family.

Walking—A Great Way to Start Moving

Walking is great—it improves fitness, strengthens muscles, helps circulation, and can relieve insomnia. It burns calories, aiding in weight loss. Daily walking can result in a positive body change. You can make it a mindful, meditative walk while you enjoy nature. In the neighborhood, it gives you a chance to get to know your neighbors.

There are a lot of benefits to walking, and it's free. Just grab your sneakers and off you go—at your own pace. To get vitamin D without exposure to the sun's strongest rays, avoid the middle of the day.

Jumping for Health

Bouncing on a rebounder, or mini trampoline, offers an amazing number of benefits. Jumping for health strengthens muscles, ligaments, and bones—and tones your internal organs, arteries, and veins. It strengthens every cell of your body with benefits from head to toe.

This non-impact aerobic exercise is suitable for everyone, although if you're overweight and concerned, consult your doctor. Also, check the weight limit for the rebounder.

A NASA study found that spending one hour on a rebounder will burn more calories than jogging for an hour. It went on to say that exercise on a mini trampoline is "the most efficient and effective exercise yet devised by man."

Some advantages to using a rebounder:

- Affordable
- Convenient
- Boosts your energy
- Weight loss
- Tones muscle
- Alkalizes your body
- Strengthens your heart and glandular system
- Relieves pain in the head, back, and neck
- Increases metabolism
- Increases performance of the heart and circulatory system
- Decreases common symptoms of the aging process

Rebounding is a unique exercise in which a weightless state is achieved at the top of each jump and landing achieves twice the force of gravity on each bounce. This shift in gravity benefits every cell of the body and provides major benefits to the lymph system. The lymphatic system typically drains at a slow pace—one to two-fifths of a teaspoon per minute. When you're bouncing on a rebounder, that number shoots up to four teaspoons per minute. This is because of the change in the gravitational pull on the body, resulting in the opening of lymphatic valves and encouraging lymphatic circulation. As you jump up, the lymphatic valves close, and as you come down, they open. The increased G-force when you land results in a rapid rise of lymphatic draining, which in turn improves circulation and detoxes the entire system. Start with small steps and bounces; then work your way up toward higher bounces. You can even bounce sitting on the rebounder. It's easy, fun, and gives the body a ton of health benefits.

S-t-r-e-t-c-h-i-n-g

Stretch daily. It keeps the muscles flexible, strong, and healthy. That flexibility is necessary to maintain a range of motion in the joints. Otherwise, muscles shorten and tighten. When you need them, they're weak and lack the ability to extend all the way. This could lead to muscle damage, joint pain, and strains.

What stretching can do for you:

- Maintain long, lean, flexible muscles
- Improve blood circulation and posture
- Reduce symptoms of disease
- Ease back pain
- Provide an overall feeling of well-being
- Activate fluids in your joints, providing more cushion so less wear from friction

If a strenuous activity suddenly stretches a tight muscle, it might become damaged. An injured muscle may be too weak to support the joints, leading to further injury. Stretching will reduce the risk of damaging a muscle or worse.

For starters, stretch your neck, shoulders, back, calves, hamstrings, hip flexors, and quadriceps. If not daily, try to do them at least three to four times a week. The goal is to maintain range of motion, regardless of your age. As with any new physical program, check with your doctor before you start.

A few things to keep in mind:

- Before stretching, warm up the muscles with a short walk or other non-strenuous activity
- Breathe—a nice deep inhale and exhale; relax and quiet your mind
- Hold the stretch steady—no movement

Strength Training

It's never too late to get active when it comes to doing strength-training exercises two to three days a week. It's important to do what you can for flexibility, balance, coordination, stamina, and strength.

Strength training helps you perform daily tasks easier and better—from standing to bending to lifting. Weights, resistance bands, and weight machines at the gym are just a few forms of strength training. Whatever you choose, you'll find a number of benefits for not only your muscles but your bones, tendons, and joints, too. Strength training helps maintain or increase the size and strength of your muscles. It can help keep you from falling and even get rid of pain. What's more, it helps maintain vitality while aging.

With weights, start out with light ones and a higher number of repetitions. Work your way up to heavier weights and lower reps. Consult the trainers at the gym, or if you're using weights at home, go online for various exercises. If you don't have dumbbells, use water bottles.

You can do body-weight strength training anywhere. Use your body weight as resistance—for example, push-ups or wall push-ups, pull-ups, squats, lunges, and crunches—with the degree of difficulty adaptable to any level of fitness. You'll build muscle and improve your core strength and range of motion in the comfort of your own home.

Resistance bands range from light to medium to heavy and extra heavy. Like bodyweight exercises, you can take your bands anywhere (even on vacation). You can find lots of different videos online for various exercises. Aim for 10 to 15 repetitions for two to three sets of each exercise.

A major reason to keep up your strength is to prevent falls. Statistics from the Centers for Disease Control (CDC) show that "falls are the leading cause of injury death in older adults and the most common cause of nonfatal injuries and hospital admissions for trauma. Falls can lead to serious injury and represent a threat to an older adult's independence."

Melissa Scott, American Council on Exercise (ACE) Certified Personal Trainer, Advanced Health and Fitness Specialist, and AARP

Affiliated Personal Trainer, said "exercises that focus on maintaining and increasing leg and core strength, such as walking on stable surfaces with varied inclines or moderately paced dance classes, along with specific exercises targeting balance, are a great combination of activities to prevent falls. Tai Chi accomplishes all of these goals, but something as simple as standing on one leg when brushing your teeth or washing dishes can help as well."

In addition to gyms, most community or senior centers, plus some libraries, offer exercise programs tailored to the needs of older adults. If you prefer to exercise at home, there are a growing number of online exercise classes that target all levels of fitness.

Another option Scott gives is to work "with a certified personal trainer with specific training and experience to suit your needs. Many trainers will meet with you in your home weekly to support you in a safe, effective workout or can meet with you a handful of times to create a home workout that meets your goals and abilities." Scott also reminds us to wear appropriate footwear and keep eyeglass prescriptions up to date to help prevent falls.

You're much less likely to fall if you stay in shape. Studies show that older adults don't recover their balance like they did when they were younger. Your brain takes a split second longer before realizing you're falling, and in that split second, momentum and gravity turn against you.

Regardless of your age and no matter what type of strength training method you use, they're all healthy and effective—if you do them.

What strength training can do for you:

- Elevate mood
- Improve sex life (need I say more?)
- More energy
- Perhaps a longer life (healthier, for sure)
- Burn calories—better weight control
- Enhance flexibility
- Reduce anxiety

- Improve muscle strength
- Boost endurance
- Sleep better
- Look better—increased self-esteem and confidence
- Help prevent disease and other health problems
- Improve quality of life

Time to get moving!

CHAPTER 14

Weighing In

RIGHT WEIGHT IS a biggie if you want to be healthy. There are too many health risks in being overweight. A healthy diet and exercise can help you reach and maintain your ideal weight. It's not something you do for six months to lose the weight and then return to your old habits. It's a lifestyle. You might be surprised just how tasty healthy eating can be. Having supportive friends and family helps.

Other ways to help keep you on track:

- A health coach
- An accountability partner
- Overeaters Anonymous

Strength and cardio exercise help keep your skin firm as you shed pounds. Muscle tissue needs to be maintained or increased to minimize loose skin.

Being overweight is a huge topic in the United States. Articles and books on dieting are popular because most American adults are overweight (two-thirds is the latest figure). To top it off, more than 30 percent of the overweight population is obese. Those extra pounds are a health hazard. Morbid obesity is the second leading preventable cause of death (cigarette smoking is the leading cause).

Morbid obesity is defined by the National Institutes of Health (NIH) as being 100 pounds or more above your ideal body weight or having a body mass index (BMI) of 40 or greater, or a BMI of 35 or more with one or more comorbidities.

During the COVID-19 pandemic, information from the CDC website said obesity increases the risk of severe illness from the virus and worsens outcomes from it. The CDC's research showed "obesity may triple the risk of hospitalization due to a COVID-19 infection" and that the vast majority of those hospitalized were obese or overweight. Yet people continue to not only overeat but to indulge in unhealthy foods, which does nothing to boost the immune system. If emotional eating is a problem when you're frustrated, angry, or anxious, working through your feelings can be helpful.

Being mindful about eating can help you watch your weight and enjoy your food. Give thanks for your meal. Avoid electronics, television, and even books while you're eating. Focus on the food and really taste it. Don't eat in a rushed manner. Put your fork down between bites. Try to chew more times than you're used to. Slowly chewing each bite at least thirty times is good for digestion as well as awareness and can help you maintain a healthy weight.

Briefly, some of the health risks of too many pounds include heart disease, heart failure, stroke, high blood pressure, gout, an increased risk for colon, breast, endometrial, and gallbladder cancers, gallbladder disease and gallstones, osteoarthritis, type 2 diabetes (formerly labeled adult-onset diabetes), and breathing problems such as sleep apnea. Type 2 diabetes is in epidemic proportion in children, so the name was changed. If you have type 2 diabetes, you can see results with good eating and exercise habits. Physical activity can have a major impact on keeping blood sugar levels down. Talk to your doctor about adjusting your insulin for exercise.

Treating all of these conditions costs billions of dollars. Estimates of the annual tab for obesity range from $90 billion to over $300 billion when including worker productivity losses, disability issues, and non-medical services. No wonder health insurance is so costly.

At work, get up from your desk and stretch, move, or take a brief walk. Take the stairs instead of the elevator. Don't wait for a close parking spot—find one from a distance and walk. While you're waiting for your plane to take off, walk around the airport.

Clinical studies vary, but being overweight and inactivity are consistently among the top health risk factors. A healthy weight is vitally important.

CHAPTER 15

Time Out

ENOUGH REST AND sleep are both important for recuperation. They relax the brain and mind and restore your body, giving it time for repair. Lack of sleep can also affect your mood. The National Sleep Foundation recommends seven to nine hours for adults. Like everything, there are exceptions. You've probably met someone, for example, who sleeps five hours a night and feels great.

A good night's sleep keeps you healthy—mentally and physically. Chronic sleep loss, sleep disorders, and deprivation can age your skin, make you forgetful, and increase stress-related disorders such as heart disease, heart attack, heart failure, high blood pressure, stomach ulcers, stroke, type 2 diabetes, and mood disorders.

A peaceful nightly routine helps shake off any tension from the day. There are ways to help you relax, unwind, and let your body and mind know it's time for sleep. You'll wake up feeling refreshed and well-rested. Keep your room dark to let the brain know it's time for sleep, and then try one or more of the suggestions listed below.

Essential Oils for Your Nightly Routine

Here are a few ways to use essential oils before bed:

- Start with a warm bath. Add six to eight drops of essential oil mixed with a carrier oil, such as almond or coconut oil, to your water. Carrier oils are used to dilute essential oils. To relax your muscles, add Epsom salt; it's also a great detoxifier.

- While you're in the tub or after you get out, use a diffuser with your choice of essential oils.
- Mix a few drops of lavender essential oil with coconut oil and massage it into your feet or dab behind your ears.
- Put a few drops of lavender on your pillowcase or on a cotton ball placed near your pillow.
- Sprinkle a few drops of essential oils with a carrier oil, such as coconut or almond, on your hands, then rub them together while you breathe in the aroma.
- In a spray bottle, add essential oil to water. Shake it up and spray around your bedroom and on your pillowcase.

Start your routine at least a half-hour before you plan to go to bed. When using essential oils, do a patch test beforehand to check for any skin sensitivity. Mix approximately one teaspoon of carrier oil with two drops of essential oil. Apply a small amount to the inside of your arm. If there's any irritation after 24 hours or so, discontinue use.

These essential oils, or a combination of them, are great choices to help you get rid of the day's stress and improve mood:

- Lavender is an all-time favorite. Its aroma is relaxing and sooth-ing, helping reduce anxiety and emotional stress and improve sleep.
- Frankincense promotes peace, relaxation, deep breathing, and spirituality. It relieves stress and lowers anxiety and feelings of being overwhelmed.
- Cedarwood and vetiver are both great options for relaxation.
- Ylang ylang assists in letting go of any frustration or anger and gives a sense of optimism.
- Bergamot helps reduce stress.
- Chamomile is calming and decreases anxiety.
- Sandalwood is grounding and promotes a feeling of inner peace.

Meditation

Meditation is covered in Chapter 10. It's a great way to start your day, but it can also help you get to sleep. There are a lot of guided meditations and meditation music, but it's best to keep electronics out of the bedroom when it's time for sleep. Try to turn them off an hour or so before retiring. Any mental activity can promote wakefulness, but even playing a relatively relaxing game on a computer or tablet device can delay sleep due to the light. If you do feel the need for listening to something, instead of earbuds, check out Sleep Phones®. They're basically small speakers inside a very comfy headband.

White noise is another tool that helps some people sleep. There are apps for this or turn on a fan or humidifier.

Breathing

If you're having trouble getting to sleep, breathing exercises can help you relax, calm the mind, and decrease stress. There are numerous other benefits to breathing exercises and entire books have been written on the breath. Two of my favorites are *The Science of Breath* by Yogi Ramacharaka and *Breath: The New Science of a Lost Art* by James Nestor. Both cover the importance of nostril breathing, which promotes deeper, fuller breaths and helps carry more oxygen throughout the body. In addition, our nasal hairs filter the air as we breathe it in. Nestor says extending inhales and exhales can impact blood pressure, mental state, and even longevity. You'll find breathing exercises in both of those books.

What's on Your Mind?

The mind seems to enjoy racing around thinking about all kinds of things when all you want to do is go to sleep. What are you thinking about as you try to drift into zzz land? A bill that's due? A meeting with the boss tomorrow? Something someone said? Take out paper and pen and write down what's on your mind or what's bothering you. It'll still be there in the morning, and you can come up with ideas or solutions during the day—or maybe even while you're sleeping.

Exercise

Physical exertion can be great in helping you sleep. It helps reduce stress and can enhance your mood. A good workout can tire you out, but best not to do it just before bedtime—otherwise, it could keep you awake. If you do want to get a little movement before sleeping, do something light like walking or stretching.

Other Sleep Tips:

- Drink a relaxing beverage like chamomile tea.
- Avoid caffeine several hours before bedtime.
- Sleep in complete darkness.
- Avoid intense television programs before heading to bed.
- Eating a light snack before bed is okay; for heavy meals, eat a few hours before you hit the hay, giving your body time to digest.
- Worry is a definite sleep buster.
- If possible, shut off the Wi-Fi signal so it doesn't interfere with your brain while you're sleeping; it'll also give your body a chance to get a deeper rest.

Rest and relaxation are just as important as sleep. Also, recreation gives your mind and body a change of pace from daily activities. By doing other pastimes, you give yourself a chance to use other areas of both the body and the brain. It's your leisure time. Do things you enjoy—movies, reading, writing, going to the beach—the list is endless. Hobbies are fun, help you de-stress, and give balance to your life. Free time spent doing things that delight you helps you unwind and sleep better. Whether you enjoy gardening, playing music, or sewing, hobbies are good for your health and mental well-being. "Me time" is an opportunity to maintain balance and feel renewed.

CHAPTER 16

Awareness

AS MENTIONED IN Chapter 11, the conscious mind comes up with an idea and sends it into the subconscious, where the idea is then carried out. So it's very important to be conscious of what thoughts and beliefs you are putting into your subconscious since those will become your experience. That's why it's a "conscious" effort to keep your focus on what you want in your life. If you do the opposite and dwell on negative thoughts long enough for them to become planted in your subconscious, you'll create an unhealthy and disappointing body and environment for yourself.

Awareness is the key. In order to stop and replace negative thoughts, we need to realize we're doing it. There are a few things you can do to help yourself become more aware. I do what's called Project Miracle, and it's had an impact on my awareness, as well as giving gratitude and having acceptance for everything just as it is. This practice is described in Melody Beattie's book, *Make Miracles in Forty Days*. You can do the project alone, but it's more fun and probably more effective with a partner. There's the accountability factor when you have a partner. For forty days, you write a list giving thanks for ten things, starting with things that bother you. For example, I'm grateful for unsolicited phone calls, the gopher holes in my yard, and my old living room carpet. You're just writing that you're thankful for them. It helps you become grateful for things just the way they are.

My miracle partner and I kept going after forty days, and we continue to do it years later. For us, the focus eventually moved from things that were bugging us to things we were truly happy to have. The exercise creates acceptance and once we accept everything, we create happiness, health, and well-being.

I find myself saying thank you a lot more and daily gratitude helps me to become more present, as well as catch negative thoughts and put a stop to them. More than ever, since starting Project Miracle, I've noticed the colors of the flowers, houses, and yards I've walked past many times and not really seen. When I'm driving, I'll notice something and say out loud, "Thank you for…" It's amazing how I can take the same route five days a week and now suddenly notice a house or a tree. Being more mindful is going to help you become more aware of every aspect of life. In turn, you'll be able to catch your not-so-pleasant thoughts when something upsetting happens. For example, getting angry when someone cuts us off in traffic only harms us, not them.

Another idea to help cultivate awareness is wearing a simple plastic bracelet. Every time you have a negative thought about someone or something, snap the bracelet and move it to the other arm. The goal is to go twenty-one days (there's that number again) without having to move it to the other arm. To be honest, I think twenty-one minutes would be great.

When I catch my thoughts going wild, I ask myself: "What about all the things you've read, the videos you've watched, the classes and seminars you've attended?" Becoming more aware is a life-long journey. You've got to be a vigilant warrior. Okay, right there I caught myself using the word warrior. No war. Another option: I practice discipline to bring peace of mind and presence. There's a big difference in vibration between the words war and peace. If the idea of words having a vibration seems odd, check out the experiments of Dr. Masaru Emoto with water crystals. Different words, such as love and hate, were placed on several jars of water which all came from the same source. After freezing the water, the crystals were examined using a microscope. Pictures of the water were taken, and it was amazing to see the difference in the water crystals. Positive words produced beautiful crystals while negative ones made ugly crystals. You can look online or watch the movie, *What the Bleep Do We Know!?*

Knowing and understanding the power of words, Mother Teresa put it this way: "I was once asked why I don't participate in anti-war demonstrations. I said that I will never do that, but as soon as you have a pro-peace rally, I'll be there."

Thoughts = feelings = vibrations = creation. What you think about, you bring about. When it comes to health, think healthy thoughts and visualize the end result you want, whether it's for you or someone else.

Summary on becoming aware:

1. Wake up and spend at least a minute or so becoming aware of your breathing. Say to yourself, "Breathe in; breathe out."
2. Give gratitude and thanks for what immediately comes to mind in the morning.
3. As you go through your day, stop once an hour to be completely present and say "Thank you" for something. I have a bracelet that vibrates every hour and reminds me to do this (http://www.meaningtopause.com). Or set your phone to go off every hour or so. It's great for a quick stretch break, too, if you sit at a computer or are in an office all day. There's a church in my neighborhood. The church bells ring three times a day. I use them to stop what I'm doing until they're done ringing.

Those are a few suggestions on becoming more aware and conscious. We will still have less-than-desirable thoughts sometimes, but now we are better equipped to catch them. If you have ways that have helped you, please share on my Facebook page Healthy by Choice, Not by Chance.

"What if..." When you start getting scenarios in your head and are concerned about something that might happen, hit the "delete"

button. Then switch your image to a positive outcome. Your image, thoughts, and feelings are powerful gifts.

Keepin' the Faith

Stories of healing often revolve around faith and belief. If you're spending your time thinking and talking about illness, disease, and how much you fear them, the results will be a lot different than focusing on faith and belief. What we feed our bodies is important but even more so is what you feed your mind. You may find that as you clean up your thoughts, you'll want to clean up your diet, too. Notice how often your mind reverts to unpleasant thoughts. Don't give up—replace them with their opposites—practice, practice, practice.

Ways to help keep a positive attitude:

- Eat healthily
- Exercise regularly
- Get plenty of sleep
- Enjoy time with friends
- Laugh
- Dance
- Spend time in nature
- Journal
- Meditate
- Turn off the news
- Listen to music that makes you feel good
- Think about something or someone that makes you smile
- Watch funny videos
- Play an instrument

I started a morning routine based on Hal Elrod's book, The Miracle Morning. He dubbed his daily practice "SAVERS":
S = Silence
A= Affirmations

V = Visualization
E = Exercise
R = Reading
S = Scribing (Writing)

It's a great way to kick-start your day on a positive note. I may not get everything done first thing in the morning; some days my reading may not happen until evening, but I do get short inspirational emails that I usually read early in the day. If you're on social media, there are groups you can join that feature feel-good quotes and thoughts.

Acceptance

Resistance to what's happening can affect your mind and body. The mind goes down a path of unwanted scenarios and the body reacts. We're resisting when we judge and criticize people and circumstances. Not resisting what happens keeps stress levels down. Feel better simply by resisting nothing. If we can't change it, the answer can be found in the Serenity Prayer:

God grant me the Serenity to accept the things I cannot change,
Courage to change the things I can, and
Wisdom to know the difference.

When our minds are on autopilot, without thinking, we judge or criticize. We can change. I keep post-it notes all over my bathroom to constantly remind me to evolve, move forward, and get rid of old habits. Dropping judgment from our lives is freeing. Everyone has permission to be true to themselves, to be who they are, whether we like who they are or not. Life is meant for love, joy, and fun. Complaining about life, as it is, is not joyful. Being okay with life, as it is, brings peace.

Here's a story about Sāi Wēng, who always kept an accepting attitude. He raised horses for a living. One day he lost a horse and his neighbor felt sorry for him, but Sāi Wēng didn't care about the horse because he didn't know if losing a horse was necessarily a bad thing. After a while, the horse returned with another beautiful horse, and the neighbor congratulated him on his good luck. But Sāi Wēng said he didn't know if it was a good or bad thing to have this new horse. His son liked the new horse a lot and often took it riding. One day his son fell off the horse and broke his leg. Again, his neighbor felt sorry for him, but Sāi Wēng said it might not be a bad thing—he would have to see. Soon war broke out, but because of his broken leg, his son couldn't go off to war like the other young men in the area. In a battle, most of the young men died.

Releasing resistance and not having attachment to the outcome allow for well-being. I remind myself that what I give out comes back to me, so I'm going to receive low-frequency vibrations when I'm putting my attention on negativity or judging others.

Accepting life as it is does not mean we never hurt or grieve. Life can be difficult. There are times of sorrow. Fill your heart with love and treat others with compassion and acceptance. These higher-frequency thoughts and actions will bless you with the positive. Appreciation and gratitude make a huge difference in life.

My morning prayer helps me get centered to do just that. It's the Third Step Prayer of Codependents Anonymous:

> *God, I give to You all that I am and all that I will be*
> *for Your healing and direction.*
> *Make new this day as I release all my worries and fears, knowing*
> *that You are by my side. Please help me to open myself to Your love,*
> *to allow Your love to heal my wounds, and to allow Your love*
> *to flow through me and from me to those around me.*
> *May Your will be done this day and always. Amen.*

CHAPTER 17

Souls Assisting Evolution

EVERYTHING IS ENERGY and is always changing—so play with it. If you're not feeling well, visualize yourself healthy.

We're like radio signals offering a frequency and the entire universe responds. Every single thing, thought, and act we perform has a vibration, a frequency. The Law of Vibration is the same as the Law of Attraction. Remember, it's a lawful and orderly universe. When you truly comprehend what that means, you begin to understand that you are 100 percent responsible for everything in your life; nothing happens outside of your creative control. There's no luck, no chance, no coincidence.

Your creations begin with you. Even if we've experienced traumatic childhoods, there is hope. We make choices and can live in the past or move forward into joy. It's okay to seek outside help. As children, we're not always equipped to deal with circumstances. As adults, though, how we react to past events now, in this present moment, is in our control. And now is all we have.

It's not that anyone is consciously creating illness or destruction or drama in their lives. It's unconscious, and that's how we spend much of our time. That's why we're practicing awareness and being present. No matter how long you practice these techniques, there are still going to be times when you're on autopilot.

Plus, there are many situations that leave us wondering how they could be "created"—injustices, abuse, violence, and discrimination, just to name a few. As an example, the seemingly senselessness of mass shootings and school shootings where many children are shot. We are looking at them as physical humans, forgetting that they are souls of the essence of the One Life. Our souls are eternal. We don't know the big, huge plans or the evolution to follow such an incident—that's infinite. Those children were physically killed, their expressions were stopped, but their essence, their Spirit, was not harmed.

To mention just one incident of several, less than 24 hours after the Sandy Hook Elementary School shooting in 2012, President Obama was on national TV with tears as he began to extol the virtue of love: "...while nothing can fill the space of a lost child or loved one, all of us can extend a hand to those in need—to remind them that we are there for them, that we are praying for them, that the love they felt for those they lost endures not just in their memories but also in ours. May God bless the memory of the victims and, in the words of Scripture, heal the brokenhearted and bind up their wounds."

These kids became a symbol of love in a world with its share of hate, greed, and corruption. One of the parents, Alissa Parker, said in an interview, "Most people know of that tragic day and the darkness that surrounded it. What they did not know is that in the aftermath, there was some good that came out of it." She spoke of a thousand acts of kindness and a miracle of healing in their hearts.

Scarlet Lewis is another mom who lost her child during that shooting. The sole effective response to the loss of her six-year-old was with love and forgiveness. She said. "When we respond with love, we take our power back. We refuse to be victims." Just six months after the shooting, on her son's 7th birthday, she chose to forgive the shooter. In honor of her son, Lewis founded The Jesse Lewis Choose Love Foundation (https://chooselovemovement.org/). The website states the Core Values:

"Nurturing, Healing Love," are the foundational values for the movement. Their individual meaning form a profound and powerful formula for choosing love:

1. Nurturing means loving kindness and gratitude.
2. Healing means forgiveness.
3. Love is compassion in action.

Can you see a little piece of God's plan? These souls assisted evolution. Everything serves a purpose. When these things take place, it changes who we are, but we are souls and isn't it possible that these events could be contributing more to the totality of Consciousness through some of these undesirable experiences? You never know God's plan until it's done—and it's never done, like the story of Sāi Wēng in the previous chapter.

We must evolve and grow. Oftentimes, we're not consciously creating. Also, some inspired teachers believe we make agreements in the non-physical before coming into this lifetime; that soul contracts, both positive and negative, were made to provide lessons and growth; that there are things we want to know and learn, and we encounter circumstances in our lives in order to obtain what we chose to accomplish during this lifetime. Souls create different roles for each other and sometimes it's through the experiences of others that we evolve and expand. That's been the case for me on many occasions. Opportunities abound for us to grow, learn, expand, and evolve.

All the world's a stage, and all the men and women merely players:
they have their exits and their entrances.
~ William Shakespeare

EPILOGUE

Free Will vs. God's Will—or Both

THE INTRODUCTION OF this book began with free will and the choices we make. Our life, our health, and body are effects; choices are the cause. The last chapter covers God's plan, God's will.

Can we have both? Free will and God's will?

I like to think so. I make choices but feel more at ease knowing that I have the Universe looking after me and covering my back.

I believe we have free will. We do have choices and make them all the time. We choose according to what's vibrating the most for us, whether positively or negatively. I believe in honesty, but if I'm hungry, would I steal food? Circumstances can totally change our choices.

And if we are all One and God is all-present, then God is everywhere. That being the case, every choice we make is of God, being we are a spark of the Divine.

I talked to a few people about their views. My sister, Bev, a student of *A Course in Miracles*, said she believes in free will, but if it's not the right choice, God's Will will prevail. She gave an example of her plan to go to Thailand. "Man plans; God laughs," she said. Although her reason for not going to Thailand was because of breast cancer, she believes, because of other circumstances, not going to Thailand probably saved her life.

Another story she shared was about a New Year's Eve. My sister is a counselor and ran into a former client at the store. The client was in recovery from drugs and alcohol. The two of them chatted for a few minutes. After the fact, her client confessed that her intention was to buy booze that night for the New Year's celebration, but upon seeing my sister, she didn't.

Sally, a fellow student and teacher of Concept Therapy, shared her view: "I personally believe that I do have a choice, that the future is a series of possibilities. Every second of every day I make a choice. Sometimes those choices change the world. Otherwise, what's the point? I find it hard to believe that a God, if there is indeed a God (since we really don't know), would create a world like ours and pre-determine every single thing in it prior to it happening. Concept Therapy not only allows you to make up your own mind, it encourages us to do so."

Michael, a certified health coach, said, "God—all powerful, all knowing, all present—sees the beginning from the end—knows the choices everyone will make and allows them to make them. He never makes robots of us by commanding us to exist in a certain way."

In my life, I strive to be better, have more compassion, more patience and be a loving, caring being. When I look back over the decades of my life, I see improvement; not always, not every day. But each day, I have a clean slate. We are not perfect, and yet we are. To me, simply because we are a speck of the Divine is perfection—as we evolve to become the most Divine little speck we can be.

I also believe in God's will and, while I can't say for sure what that is, I'm thinking it's all about evolution—that we evolve to become better and better versions of ourselves.

Every day, in every way, I am getting better and better."
~Émile Coué

ACKNOWLDEGEMENTS

MANY THANKS TO you for reading my words. My hope is that some of them will resonate, inspire, motivate, or help you in some way.

A heart full of love, joy, and gratitude to my family, all such amazing teachers: my two kids, Caleb and Kaipo, who have taught me some of my biggest lessons; my parents and my siblings who helped mold me in my early childhood days and continue to guide me—Barb, Bev, Beth, and Tim.

My deepest appreciation to my dear friend, Cindy Wood. Your amazing skills help me improve as a writer. Thanks for always looking over my words, offering suggestions, editing, and being the beautiful, kind soul you are.

Love and gratitude for the ongoing support as I worked on this book from my soul sister, Lisa Winston, my miracle partner, Jane Asher, my holistic advisor and healer, Claire Levy, and my mentor, Dr. Frank. I'm grateful for your feedback, time, help, motivating words, and most of all, your love and friendship.

Thank you, Louise Mathews, for your willingness to share your expertise as I wrapped up the writing of this book and was ready to get it published.

Appreciation to Kevin Bradley and Susan Paton, for your editing expertise.

A big thank you to the kind and helpful experts at Outskirts Press for taking my manuscript and turning it into a book you can see, feel, touch, and hold.

Many thanks to so many who have blessed me with their wisdom and knowledge.

Love, health, and happiness to all.

ABOUT THE AUTHOR

JO EAGER IS an award-winning international broadcast and print journalist, reporter, and writer. Her voice aired around the world—from former East Germany to Kauai, Hawaii, and several places in between—in English and German. She has broadcast from studios, a Cessna, and a helicopter.

As a teenager, she began working at a radio station as a copywriter and disc jockey. Since then, several of her stories have appeared in *Chicken Soup for the Soul* books, along with hundreds of articles published in magazines, newspapers, and online: *USA Today, Just Labs, California Game and Fish, San Diego Union-Tribune, San Francisco Examiner, Girlfriends, Sacramento Bee, Well & Healthy Woman, Kauai Times*, and *Curves*, among many others.

A student of universal laws, nutrition, and fitness, and a passion for health and well-being, Jo shares lessons learned through challenges in her life and her children's—a life-threatening rattlesnake bite, helicopter crash, autoimmune disorder, and gender identity.

A veteran of the U.S. Army, she served at the American Forces Network in Berlin, Germany, which at that time was 101 miles behind the Iron Curtain and surrounded by the Berlin Wall. She later worked in the German language at Radio in the American Sector, formed after WWII to broadcast from the west into the east during the Cold War.

Jo assisted *USA Today* and several U.S. radio stations with coverage of the fall of the Berlin Wall.

Based in San Diego, Jo freelances as a writer, voice actor, fitness instructor, and commercial and background actor.

WHERE TO FIND JO EAGER ONLINE

Website: jo-eager.com

Facebook Personal: https://www.facebook.com/jo.eager.16/

Facebook Book Fan page:
https://www.facebook.com/HealthyChoicesMindBodySoul

LinkedIn: https://www.linkedin.com/in/jo-eager-a22b688/

Instagram: https://www.instagram.com/jo.eager/

Twitter: https://twitter.com/eagerwriter

YouTube Channel:
https://www.youtube.com/channel/UCYpjQOe7X-w3CG41vg0SiKw

CPSIA information can be obtained
at www.ICGtesting.com
Printed in the USA
BVHW050049290423
663236BV00004B/15